ÖSTERREICHISCHE AKADEMIE DER WISSENSCHAFTEN
PHILOSOPHISCH-HISTORISCHE KLASSE
SITZUNGSBERICHTE, 811. BAND

VERÖFFENTLICHUNGEN ZUR IRANISTIK
HERAUSGEGEBEN VON BERT G. FRAGNER UND VELIZAR SADOVSKI

NR. 55

ELA FILIPPONE

THE FINGERS AND THEIR NAMES IN THE IRANIAN LANGUAGES

(Onomasiological Studies on Body-Part Terms, I)

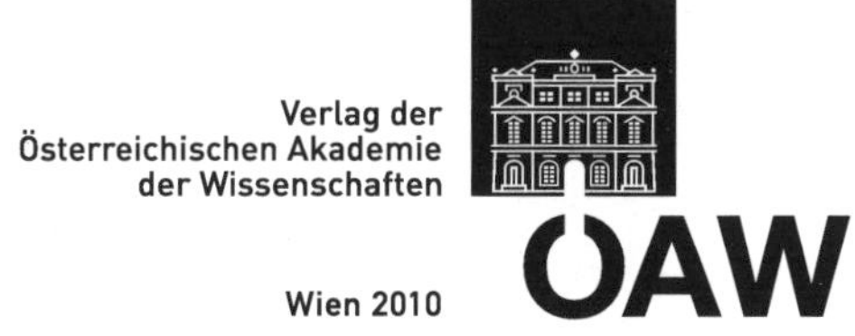

Wien 2010

Vorgelegt von w. M. Bert G. Fragner
in der Sitzung am 13. März 2009

British Library Cataloguing in Publication data
A Catalogue record of this book is available from the British Library

Die verwendete Papiersorte ist aus chlorfrei gebleichtem Zellstoff hergestellt, frei von säurebildenden Bestandteilen und alterungsbeständig.

ISBN 978-3-7001-6657-3

Druck: Druckerei Ferdinand Berger & Söhne Ges.m.b.H., A-3580 Horn

Printed and bound in the EU

http://hw.oeaw.ac.at/6657-3
http://verlag.oeaw.ac.at

CONTENTS

PREFACE

This work is a part of a broader project that I planned years ago in the frame of the *Ethnolinguistics of the Iranian area Project*, directed by Adriano V. Rossi for over fifteen years (funded by the Italian Ministry for Scientific Research, last code no. 9710425417). My task was to collect and describe the Iranian body part terminology in a cross-linguistic perspective and with a motivational approach, contributing in this way to a better knowledge of the Iranian lexicon in a comparativistic view. For this purpose, I have been collecting for years words and expressions relevant to the anatomical lexicon from ancient and modern Iranian languages, mostly using as sources published dictionaries, glossaries and running texts, and for some languages, mainly Balochi, but also Persian, Baxtiāri, Kurdish, Ossetic etc., spoken texts recorded by me and other scholars, working with native speakers. The data-base produced so far contains several thousands of words and appears to be of remarkable interest, considering that a great amount of native lexicography – often difficult to trace in Europe – has been included into the analysis.

The first step of this project was the publication in 1995 of *The pupil of the eye in the Iranian languages* in the series *Etnolinguistica dell'area iranica*, Naples. The present book, in which the words for 'finger' and the names of every single finger in the Iranian languages are surveyed, is the second one. Hopefully, further issues will be published in the near future.

The idea to concentrate on the finger lexical domain in Iranian originated from a research conducted in Balochistan with the help of many Balochi speakers in the 1980s, whose results have been published in a provisional version in the early 1990s and in its definitive version (with considerable delay) as FILIPPONE 2000–2003.

A draft of the present study was more or less completed around 2000. For several reasons I preferred to let it decant for some years before its publication. This settling period proved to be useful because in the meantime a relevant amount of fresh material was added to that already recorded, also thanks to recent publications, especially from Iran, where dialectology has been receiving increasing attention and interest. Moreover, I had the opportunity to add important suggestions coming from many scholars on single items.

A preliminary presentation of a few results of this research was done on the occasion of the first Italo-Austrian Iranological meeting held in Cagli (17–19 september 2005), at the beautiful library of Prof. Gherardo Gnoli's private residence, when a more strict cooperation between the Italian scholars active in Iranian philology and the scholars of the Institut für Iranistik of the Austrian Academy of Sciences started up. To me, that meeting was a chance to develop productive and pleasant scientific relations with new colleagues, and also warm friendship with some of the members of the Institute, in particular Prof. Bert Fragner and Doz. Velizar Sadovski. It was there that the idea originated of publishing the present essay in the framework of the *Veröffentlichungen zur Iranistik* of the Academy, as a first issue of a project of several volumes under the general title "Onomasiological Studies on Body-Part Terms".

Scholars and friends to whom I have applied during the years and who have contributed in different ways to this publication, are many. I would wish to mention here (in alphabetical order) at least the most involved: Dr Sabir Badalkhan; Prof. Paolo Calvetti (for Japanese); Prof. Mauro Maggi; Dr Enrico Morano; Prof. ʿAli Ašraf Sādeqi; Prof. Martin Schwartz; Prof. Werner Sundermann. To Prof. Hasan Rezāi Bāγbidi I am particularly grateful for his important contribution both as a scholar and as a Persian native speaker. Many cordial thanks are due to Prof. Rüdiger Schmitt, who read a preliminary draft of this work, and kindly provided me with precious suggestions and annotations. I also remember with gratitude and love the kindness with which Prof. Ilya Gershevitch read (almost twenty years ago) a preliminary study on the Balochi finger names. Special thanks are due to the Italian young researchers working on Iranian dialectology, Dr Gerardo Barbera, Dr Matteo De Chiara and Dr Daniele Guizzo, all of them having generously placed at my disposal their unpublished data on Minābi/Baškardi, Pashto and Tāleši respectively. I am much indebted to my dear friend Velizar Sadovski for all that he has done as editor of the series, responsible for the volume, on our meetings both in Austria and in Italy.

I want to thank all my Balochi friends, which I always remember with affection. I also want to express my gratitude to my Ossetian friends; my thought runs in particular to the late Vitaly Gussalov, whose untimely death deeply saddened all Italian friends of Ossetia. Heartful thanks also go to all my occasional Iranian and Pakistani informants. They have been many, and I cannot mention all. I will quote by name only one of them, Mr Ebrahim Širāzi, a Shirazi taxi-driver who volunteered to help me in my research, personally asking the finger names to people who crowded a bookshop at Shiraz. The data elicited on that occasion resulted of no particular interest, but his enthusiastic willingness in helping me was really moving, and I consider

Mr Širāzi's kindness as emblematic of the friendly attitude of many people I met during my research in Iran and Pakistan.

Last, but not least I have to acknowledge uninterrupted suggestions and support by Adriano V. Rossi, my former tutor in Iranian philology and (subsequently) my husband. Working alongside him is for me an unwavering source of joy.

This book is dedicated to the memory of my father, Francesco Paolo Filippone.

The main problems I faced with in my research are those typical of all extensive works (typological and universalistic), and concern the nature of the available sources. The unevenness in the linguistic documentation used is striking, but unavoidable. For some of the Iranian languages involved in the survey, data have been collected through interviews, questionnaires and recordings of spontaneous speech, mainly ordinary fieldwork conversations with a large number of native speakers; however, the documentation concerning the majority of the languages (both ancient and modern) results from desk work, through sorting dictionaries, glossaries and texts. Unfortunately, data extrapolated from dictionaries rarely can be considered as exhaustive. This is of course due to the uneven quality of the available lexicographical works. For some languages, we can rely on research traditions and comprehensive descriptions, which allow for a shared understanding of the relevant linguistic systems at a diachronic level, and also provide precious insights into the cultural, historical, religious etc. frameworks. For other languages, systematic studies are completely wanting. Some languages have a long written tradition, some others do not. Furthermore, a series of terms pertaining to colloquial registers are commonly not recorded at all even in major dictionaries for different reasons (including taboos). It should be added that data retrieved from lexicographical repertoires are to be considered with great care because contexts, transmitters of the message and in general the sociolinguistic categories of usage are often completely disregarded, and the diachronic dimensions are levelled. It follows that in most dictionaries, terms no more existing in a particular language or restricted to a particular stylistic level and condition are mixed up with terms of common use. The consequence is that I had no possibility of examining the collected data according to a contextualized, pragmatic conception of onomasiology, which focuses on the actual choises made for a particular term as a designation of a particular referent.[1]

Nevertheless, I still think that some inaccuracies in the details do not generally invalidate the results achieved in identifying associative patterns active in the denomination processes. I hope, therefore, that the amplitude of the lexical data here gathered and commented on can somehow manage to counterbalance the mentioned inconsistencies of the sources.

Another crucial problem for works like the present one is that of the transcription systems. Some of the languages taken into consideration have a long written tradition, as is the case with Persian, whose writing system, the Arabo-Persian script, has been in use for centuries. To let gain access to readers who are not specialists in Iranian languages, and are not accustomed to that alphabet, Persian words have been quoted in a phonemic transcription (*not* transliteration), according to the modern standard pronunciation of Iran. I followed in the main the lines of LAZARD's (1990a) transcription, which is tendentially phonemic. Some minor modifications have been introduced; in particular (1) ق transcribed *q* and غ transcribed *γ* (though the problem of the phonemic status of the uvular voiceless stop and the corresponding voiced fricative in the modern standard of Iran seems nowadays mostly settled in favour of one single phoneme); (2) the mid-back vowel transcribed *ā* (LAZARD: *â*).

A tendentially phonemic transcription has also been used for Balochi. To avoid misunderstandings, I preferred following the traditional praxis of opposing tense vowels to lax ones, differentiating the two sets by means of a macron (*ī*, *ū*, *ā* ~ *i*, *u*, *a*), instead of using the IPA symbols ([i], [u], [a] ~ [ɪ], [ʊ], [ə]) according to the guidelines of the *Balochi Comparative Etymological Dictionary Project* (Department of Asian Studies, L'Orientale University, Naples).

For all the other Iranian languages, I have stuck where possible to the systems used by the individual authors of the written sources from which any single expression has been extrapolated. In a few cases, minor phonetic details have not been reproduced. As a downside of this procedure, it follows that it could be possible to find two quotations of the same word from a given language with different transcriptions because different sources, with different approaches and traditions, have been used. In case of ambiguity, the reader has to go back up to the original source, which is always (directly or indirectly) retrievable. When a quoted word is not followed by the reference to its source, this means that the source in question is considered as the

---

[1] For a use-oriented conception of onomasiology, see GRONDELAERS – GEERAERTS 2003.

"main one" for that given language, being mentioned once and for all in the list of language/dialect abbreviations (see p. 11). The choice of the "main source" for a language is only based on the amount of terms selected for the present investigation and here quoted, and it does not imply an evaluation of any particular work. In source references, the number of page is not given when the work from which the quoted word is taken, is (or contains a section which is) alphabetically ordered, and this concerns dictionaries, glossaries or any kind of works provided with a lexical list. The glosses defining Iranian words extrapolated from dictionaries whose target language is other than English, are generally translated into English; the original gloss is added only when relevant to the discussion of a particular term and/or considered useful in order to avoid misunderstanding.

An especially burning question, also implying sociolinguistic and ideological problems, is represented by the means of transcribing the different forms subsumed under the cover term 'Kurdish'. The Kurdish varieties have different writing traditions, using different alphabets (with several subvariants). Kurdish items taken out from dictionaries using the more or less standardised Roman-based orthography originally developed by the Bedir-Khan brothers in the 1930s or phonetically more detailed variants of this orthography (mostly northern and central dialects) are quoted according to the spelling adopted by each author. Kurdish items taken out from dictionaries using Arabo-Persian script (mostly southern varieties: HAŽĀR 1990, SAFIZĀDE 2001, etc.) are transcribed according to the lines commonly adopted by Iranian scholars. Therefore readers must be extremely careful. Note in particular the opposition *ā* : *a* in Southern Krd. (quoted in transcription from Ar.-Prs. writing) as contrasted with the opposition *a* : *e* in Northern / Central Krd. (quoted in its traditional Roman alphabet). Note also Southern Krd. *ǰ* = Northern / Central Krd. *c*, Southern Krd. *č* =Northern / Central Krd. *ç*.

ABBREVIATIONS

Languages / Dialects[2]

Adb.	Abdui (Krd. dial.)	Salāmi 2004 (64, 174)
Abiā.	Abiānei	Lecoq 2002
AfγPrs.	Persian of Afghanistan	Afγāni Nevis 1956
Her.	Herati	Āsef Fekrat 1997
Kāb.	Kābuli	
Aft.	Aftari	Homāyun 1992b
AliĀb.	See Māz.	
Āmol.	See Māz.	
Āmor.	Āmorei	ᶜĀdelxāni 2000
Anār.	Anāraki	Sohrābi Anāraki 1994
Ar.	Arabic	Wehr 1979
Arāk.	Arāki	Mohtāt n.d.
Ār.-Bidg.	Ārāni – Bidgoli	ᶜAlijānzāde 1993
Ardest.	Ardestāni	Lecoq 2002
Āšt.	Āštiāni	Moqdam 1949: 33, 80
Av.	Avestan	Bartholomae 1904
Gath.	Gathic	
Āvarz.	Āvarzamāni	Dehghan 1970
Awr.	See Gorāni	
Bactr.	Bactrian	
Badaxš.	Badaxšāni	Lorimer 1922
Bādr.	Bādrudi	Lecoq 2002
Baǰ.	Baǰoi	Karamšoev 1988 – 1991 – 1999
Bal.	Balochi	my own data; Archive of the Balochi Comparative Etymological Dictionary Project, Naples – Rome
EBal.	Eastern Balochi	
SBal.	Southern Balochi	
WBal.	Western Balochi	
Baliā.	Baliāni	Salāmi 2006 (58, 188)
Ban.	Banāfi	Salāmi 2005 (66, 176)
Bard.	Bardesiri	Barumand Saʿid 1991
Bart.	Bartangi	
Bast.	Bastaki	Bastaki 1980
Birǰ.	Birǰandi	Rezāi 1994
Birov.	Birovakāni	Salāmi 2006 (58, 188)
Biz.	Bizovoi (Abuzeydābādi)	Lecoq 2002
Bohr.	Bohrui	Žukovskij 1888
BoirAhm.	See Lo.	

[2] Names of languages/dialects with a (more or less strong) tradition in English are spelled according to that tradition. Otherwise, they appear in transcription or in a broad transcription (i.e., only partially diacriticised), as the result of several compromises: normalization in this matter is all but impossible. The third column refers to the main source (if any) for each Iranian language/dialect; see above p. 8.

Br.	Brahui	ROSSI 1979
Bšk.	Baškardi	
NBšk.	North Baškardi	
SBšk.	South Baškardi	
Buš.	Bušehri	HAMIDI 2001
Bxt.	Baxtiāri	SĀLEHI 1990
ČLang	Čahār Lang	SARLAK 2002
Pāgač	Pāgač	KALAKI 1973
ČLang	See Bxt.	
Dādenǰ.	Dādenǰāni	SALĀMI 2006 (58, 188)
Dahl.	Dahlei	SALĀMI 2004 (64, 176)
Damāv.	Damāvandi	ᶜALAMDĀRI 2005
Dāreng.	Dārengāni (Lor, Fārs)	SALĀMI 2006 (59, 189)
Dašt.	Daštestāni	BORAZJĀNI 2003
Dav.	Davāni	SALĀMI 2002
Del.	(Rāǰi) Deliǰāni	SAFARI 1994
Dezf.	Dezfuli	EMĀM 2000
Dežg.	Dežgāhi	SALĀMI 2006 (59, 189)
Dig.	See Oss.	
Dorun.	Dorunaki / Mehbudi	SALĀMI 2006 (59, 189)
Drav.	Dravidian	
Dusir.	Dusirāni	SALĀMI 2005 (66, 176)
Dzadr.	See Pšt.	
Engl.	English	
Esf-JPrs.	See JPrs.	
Esf.Prs.	Persian of Esfahān	KALBĀSI 1991
Farām.	Farāmarzi	FARĀMARZI 1984
Fin.	Fini	NAJIBI FINI 2002
Frv.	Farvi	FRYE 1949
Gahw.	See Gorāni	
Garr.	See Kurdish	
Gath.	See Avestan	
Ger.	See Lārest.	
Gil.	Gilaki	MARᶜAŠI 2003
Māč.	Māčiāni	FARZPUR MĀČIĀNI 1954–1955
Rams.	Rāmsari	ŠOKRI 2006
Gor.	Gorāni	
Awr.	Awromāni	MACKENZIE 1966
Gahw.	Gahwārai	HADANK 1930
Kand.	Kandulai	HADANK 1930
Gorgn.	Gorganāi	SALĀMI 2005 (67, 177, 179)
Gr.	Greek	LIDDELL – SCOTT 1996
Gz.	Gazi	EILERS 1979
Ham.	Hamadāni	GARUSIN 1991
Hanǰ.	Hanǰani	ĀQĀRABIᶜ 2004
Her.	See AfγPrs.	
Hay.	Hayāti	SALĀMI 2006 (58, 188)
Haz.	Hazaragi	TĀRIQ MĀLISTĀNI 1993
Horm.	Hormuzi (Banderi)	SKJÆRVØ 1975
IA	Indo-Aryan	

IE	Indo-European	
IIr.	Indo-Iranian	
Ir.	Iranian	
IrĀz.	Āzari (Ir. dialects)	
Čā.	Čāli	YARSHATER 2001 (280–289)
Ebr.	Ebrāhimābādi	ĀL-E AHMAD 1959
Ešt.	Eštehārdi	
Harz.	Harzani	KĀRENG 1954
Ker.	Keringāni	ZOKĀ 1954
Sagz.	Sagzābādi	ĀL-E AHMAD 1959
Xoi.	Xoini	SOTUDE 1958 (325)
Išk.	Iškāšmi	PAXALINA 1959
It.	Italian	
Jawš.	Jawšaqāni	LAMBTON 1938
Jir.	Jirofti	DEHQĀNI 1998
JPrs.	Judeo-Persian	
Esf-JPrs.	Judeo-Persian of Esfahān	KALBĀSI 1994
Ham-JPrs	Judeo-Persian of Hamādan	ABRAHAMIAN 1936
Yzd-JPrs.	Judeo-Persian of Yazd	HOMĀYUN 2004
Kāb.	See AfγPrs.	
Kafr.	Kafrāni	ŽUKOVSKIJ 1922 (110)
Kah.	Kahaki	MOQDAM 149 (33, 80)
Kahn.	Kahnuǰi	DEHQĀNI 1998)
Kal. (Lor)	Kalāni (Lor) (Kaluni)	SALĀMI 2004 (65, 175)
Kal. (Tāǰ.)	Kalāni (Tāǰiki)	SALĀMI 2005 (67, 177)
Kand.	See Gorāni	
Kāz.	Kāzeruni	SALĀMI 2004 (64, 174)
Kelār.	See Māz.	
Kerm.	Kermāni	PURHOSEINI 1991
ZorKerm.	Zoroastrian Kermāni	SORUŠIĀN 1956
Keš.	Kešei	ŽUKOVSKIJ 1888
Khot.	Khotanese	BAILEY 1979
Khwar.	Khwarezmian	BENZING – TARAF 1983
Knd.	Kandei	SALĀMI 2004 (65, 175)
Kor.	Koruni	SALAMI 2006 (59, 189)
Krd.	Kurdish	
Garr.	Garrusi	CHRISTENSEN – BARR 1939
Krmnš.	Kirmânšâhî	DARVIŠIĀN 1996
KurmKrd.	Kurmanji	CHYET 2003
Mahâb.	Mahâbâdî	KALBĀSI 1983
SouthKrd.	Southern Kurdish	HAŽĀR 1990
SulKrd.	Sulêmanî	WAHBY – EDMONDS 1966
Korš.	Koroši (Bal. dial.)	SALĀMI 2006 (59, 189)
Kuhp.	Kuhpāyi	EILERS 1990
Kumz.	Kumzāri	THOMAS 1930
Kuz.	Kuzargi	SALĀMI 2004 (65, 175)
Lak.	Lakki	IZADPANĀH 1989
Lār.	see Lārest.	
Lārest.	Lārestāni	EQTEDĀRI 1955
Ger.	Gerāši	

Lār.	Lāri	
Lāsg.	Lāsgerdi	SOTUDE 1963
Lat.	Latin	
Lir.-Dayl.	Lirāvi – Daylami	LIRĀVI 2001
Lo.	Lori	IZADPANĀH 2001
BoirAhm.	Boir Ahmadi	LAMᶜE 1970
Bālā-Gar.	Bālā Garive	AMANOLAHI – THACKSTON 1986
Madagl.	Madaglašti	LORIMER 1922
Mah.	Mahallāti	
Mahâb.	see Krd.	
Mamas.	Mamassani (Lori)	SALĀMI 2004 (65, 175)
Māč	See Gilaki	
Mās.	Māsarmi	SALĀMI 2004 (65, 175)
Māz.	Māzandarāni	NAJAFZĀDE-YE BĀRFORUŠ 1989
AliĀb.	Ali Ābādi	SOTUDE 1962
Āmol.	Āmoli	PARTAVI ĀMOLI 1979
Kelār.	Kelārdašti	KALBĀSI 1997
Sār.	Sāri	ŠOKRI 1995
Mei.	Meimei	LAMBTON 1938
Min.	Minābi (Banderi)	BARBERA 2004
MIr.	Middle Iranian	
Mnǰ.	Munǰi	GRJUNBERG 1972
Mosq.	Mosqāni	SALĀMI 2005 (67, 177)
MPrs.	Middle Persian	
Phl.	Pahlavi	MACKENZIE 1971
Man. MPrs.	Manichaean MPrs.	DURKIN-MEISTERERNST 2004
Nāi.	Nāini	SOTUDE 1986
Nat.	Natanzi	ŽUKOVSKIJ 1888: 63–64
Nud.	Nudāni	SALĀMI 2005 (67, 177)
NWIr.	North Western Iranian	
OIr.	Old Iranian	
Ōrm.	Ōrmuṛi	IIFL-I
Oroš.	Orošori (Rošorvi)	
Oss.	Ossetic	IESOJ
Dig.	Digor	
Pāp.	Pāpuni	SALĀMI 2005 (66, 176)
Par.	Parāči	KIEFFER 1979–1980
Phl.	see MPrs.	
Pol.	Polish	
Prs.	Persian	FF
Prth.	Parthian	
Man. Prth.	Manichaean Parthian	DURKIN-MEISTERERNST 2004
Pšt.	Pashto	ASLANOV 1966
Dzadr.	Dzadrāni	SEPTFONDS 1994
Wan.	Wanetsi	ELFENBEIN 1967
Qāi.	Qāini	ZOMORRODIĀN 1989
Qasr.	Qasrāni	DEYHIM 2005
Qm.	Qomi	SĀDEQI 2001
Qohr.	Qohrudi	LECOQ 2002
Rāv.	Rāvari	KARBĀSI RĀVARI 1987

Rič.	Riči	SALĀMI 2005 (66, 176)
Rod.	Rodāni	MOᶜTAMEDI 2001
Roš.	Rošani	SOKOLOVA 1959
Russ.	Russian	
Sang.	Sangesari	SOTUDE 1963
Sār.	see Māz.	
Sariq.	Sariqōli	PAXALINA 1971
Sarv.	Sarvestāni	HOMĀYUN 1992a
Sed.	Sedei	ŽUKOVSKIJ 1922: 110
Semn.	Semnāni	SOTUDE 1963
Sgd.	Sogdian	GHARIB 1995
Sgl.	Sangleči	IIFL-II
Si.	Sindhi	PARMĀNAND MĒWĀRĀM 1910
Sir.	Siraiki	JUKES 1961
Sirǰ.	Sirǰāni	SARYAZDI 2001
Sist.	Sistāni	MOHAMMADI XOMAK 2000
Siv.	Sivandi	EILERS 1988
Skt.	Sanskrit	MONIER-WILLIAMS 1899
Somγ.	Somγāni	SALĀMI 2005 (67, 177)
SouthKrd.	see Krd.	
Srx.	Sorxei	SOTUDE 1963
Sul.	see Krd.	
Šahm.	Šahmirzādi	SOTUDE 1963
Šγn.	Šuγni	KARAMŠOEV 1988 – 1991 – 1999
Šir.	Širāzi	BEHRUZI 1969
Šušt	Šuštari	NIRUMAND 1976
SWIr.	South Western Iranian	
Tafr.	Tafreši	
Taj.	Tajik	FZT
Tāl.	Tāleši	PIREJKO 1976
Talahed.	Talahedeški	ŽUKOVSKIJ 1922: 110
Tār.	Tāri	LECOQ 2002
Tehr.	Tehrāni	
TrbHayd.	Turbat Haydarie	DĀNEŠGAR 1995
Turk.	Turkish	REDHOUSE 1968
TurkĀz.	(Turkish) Āzeri	BEHZĀDI 1990
Ur.	Urdu	PLATTS 1930
Varz.	Varzenei	LECOQ 2002
Vfs.	Vafsi	STILO 2004
Voniš.	Vonišuni	ŽUKOVSKIJ 1888: 63–64
Wan.	see Pšt.	
Wx.	Waxi	GRJUNBERG – STEBLIN-KAMENSKIJ 1976
Xor.	Xorāsāni	ŠĀLČI 1991
Xuf.	Xufi	SOKOLOVA 1959
Xuns.	Xunsāri	AŠRAFI XĀNSĀRI 2004
Xur.	Xuri	ŠĀYEGĀN 2006
Yγn.	Yaγnobi	ANDREEV – PEŠČEREVA 1957
Yzd.	Yazdi	
ZorYzd.	Zoroastrian Yazdi	VAHMAN – ASATRIAN 2002 (p. 59)

Ydγ.	Yidγa	IIFL-II
Yzγ.	Yazγulāmi	ĖDEL'MANN 1971
Zā.	Zāzā	PAUL 1998
Zar.	Zarandi	BĀBAK 1996
Zarq.	Zarqāni	MALEKZĀDE 2001
Zefr.	Zefrei	ŽUKOVSKIJ 1888: 63–64
ZorKerm.	see Kerm.	
ZorYzd.	see Yzd.	

BIBLIOGRAPHICAL ABBREVIATIONS

CDIAL	see TURNER 1966
COD	see FOWLER – FOWLER 1919
DBIA	EMENEAU – BURROW 1962
DED[2]	BURROW – EMENEAU 1984
DEHX	see DEHXODĀ 1946-1981
EVP	see MORGENSTIERNE 1927
EVŠG	see MORGENSTIERNE 1974
EWA	see MAYRHOFER
FF	see MOᶜIN 1371/1992
FZT	*Farhang-i Zabon-i Tojiki*
IESOJ	see Abaev
IEW	see POKORNY 1959
IIFL I	see MORGENSTIERNE 1929
IIFL II	see MORGENSTIERNE 1938
KEWA	MAYRHOFER
NEVP	see MORGENSTIERNE 2003

OTHER ABBREVIATIONS

Dk.	*Dēnkard*
FrO	*Frahang ī Ōīm*
GrBd.	*Greater Bundahišn*
Nēr.	*Nērangistān*
p.c.	personal communication
PRdD.	*Pahlavi Rivāyat Accompanying the Dādestān ī Dēnīg*
Vd.	*Vīdēvdād* (*Vendidad*)
Y.	*Yasna*
Yt.	*Yašt*
WZ	*Wizīdagīhā ī Zādsprām*

BIBLIOGRAPHY

ABDOLI 2001 = ABDOLI, [c]A.: *Farhang-e tatbiqi-e tāleši, tāti, āzari*. Tehrān 1380/2001.

ABDURAXMANOV 1954 = ABDURAXMANOV, R.: *Russko-uzbekskij slovar': 50000 slov; s pril. grammatičeskix tablič russkogo jazyka*. Moskva 1954.

[c]ABDUL QAYYŪM BALOČ 1997 = [c]ABDUL QAYYŪM BALOČ: *Baločī būmyā*. Qoeṭṭa 1997.

ABRAHAMIAN 1936 = ABRAHAMIAN, R.: *Dialectes des israélites de Hamadan et d'Ispahan et dialecte de Baba Tahir*. (Dialectologie iranienne). Paris 1936.

ABRAMJAN 1965 = ABRAMJAN, R.: *Pexlevijsko-persidsko-armjano-russko-anglijskij slovar'*. Erevan 1965.

[c]ĀDELXĀNI 2000 = [c]ĀDELXĀNI, H.: *Farhange Āmorei (vāženāme, farhang-e emsāl va kenāyāt va ..). Jeld-e avval*. Arāk 1379/2000.

ADIB TUSI 1963–1964 = ADIB TUSI, M. A: 'Farhang-e loγāt-e bāzyāfte (mostadarak)', *Našrie-ye dāneškade-ye adabiāt-e Tabriz*, 15/3, 15/4 (1342/1963); 16/1, 16/2, 16/3 (1343/1964).

ADIB TUSI 1992 = ADIB TUSI, M. A.: 'Namune-ye čand az loγāt-e āzari', in AFŠĀR, I. (ed.), *Zabān-e fārsi dar Āzerbāiǰān* II. *Az neveštehā-ye dānešmandān va zabānšenāsān*. Tehrān 1371/1992, 235–361 [first publ. in *Našrie-ye Dāneškade-ye adabiāt-e Tabriz* 8–9 (1335/1956 – 1336/1957)].

AFΓĀNI NEVIS 1956 = AFΓĀNI NEVIS, [c]A.: *Loγāt-e [c]āmiāne-ye fārsi-ye Afγānistān*. Afγānistān 1335/1956.

AFŠĀR 1989 = AFŠĀR, I.: *Vāženāme-ye yazdi*. (Selsele-ye matun-e va tahqiqāt az entešārāt-e ǰedāgāne-ye Farhang-e Irān Zamin 35 – Ganǰine-ye Hosein-e Bašārat barā-ye pežuheš dar farhang va tārix-e Yazd 2) Tehrān 1368/1989.

AFŠĀR SISTĀNI 1986 = AFŠĀR SISTĀNI, I.: *Vāženāme-ye sistāni*. (Bonyād-e Nišāpur 13). Tehrān 1365/1986.

[c]ALAMDĀRI 2005 = [c]ALAMDĀRI, M.: *Guyeš-e damāvandi*. (Pežuhešgāh-e [c]olum-e ensāni va motālehāt-e farhangi). Tehrān 1374/2005.

ĀL-E AHMAD 1959 = ĀL-E AHMAD, J.: *Tātnešinhā-ye Boluk-e Zahrā*. Tehrān 1337/ 1959 (repr. 1353/1974).

'ALIJĀNZĀDE 1993 = 'ALIJĀNZĀDE, H.: *Zabān-e Kavir. Ketāb-e avval: Tahqiq dar zabān-e Ārān va Bidgol*. N.p. 1372/1993.

ALINEI 1996 = ALINEI, M.: 'Aspetti teorici della motivazione', *Quaderni di semantica* XVII (1996), 7–17.

ALINEI 2009 = ALINEI, M.: 'Le origini linguistiche e antropologiche della filastrocca', *Quaderni di semantica* XXX (2009), 263–289.

AMANOLAHI – THACKSTON 1986 = AMANOLAHI, S. – THACKSTON, W. M.: *Tales from Luristan* (*Matalyâ Lurissʉ*). (Harvard Iranian Series 4). Harvard 1986.

AMÎRXAN 1992 = AMÎRXAN: *Kurdisch-Deutsch (Teil 1) – Deutsch-Kurdisch (Teil 2)*. Ismaning 1992.

AMOUZGAR – TAFAZZOLI 2000 = AMOUZGAR, J. – TAFAZZOLI, A.: *Le cinquième livre du Dēnkard*. (Studia Iranica – Cahier 23). Paris 2000.

ANDRÉ 1991 = ANDRÉ, J. : *Le vocabulaire latin de l'anatomie*. (Collection d'études anciennes 59. Série latine). Paris 1991.

ANDREEV – PEŠČEREVA 1957 = ANDREEV, M. S. – PEŠČEREVA, E. M.: *Jagnobskie teksty*. Moskva – Leningrad 1957.

ANKLESARIA 1949 = ANKLESARIA, B. T.: *Pahlavi Vendidâd. Transliteration and translation in English* (ed. by D. D. Kapadia). Bombay 1949.

ANKLESARIA 1956 = ANKLESARIA, B. T.: *Zand – Ākāsīh. Iranian or Greater Bundahišn*. Bombay 1956.

ANJOM ŠO^{c}Ā^c 2002 = ANJOM ŠO^{c}Ā^c, M.: *Rāyeǰtarin estelāhāt va guyeshā-ye Kermān*. Kermān 1381/2002.

ANONBY 2003 = ANONBY, E. J.: 'Update on Luri: How many languages?', *Journal of the Royal Asiatic Society*. 3rd Series. 3, 13/2 (2003), 171–197.

ANUŠE 1997 = ANUŠE, H.: *Farhangnāme-ye adabi-e fārsi. Dānešnāme-ye adab-e fārsi. J̌eld-e dovvom*. Tehrān 1376/1997.

ĀQĀRABI^c 2004 = ĀQĀRABI^c, A.: *Guyeš-e rāǰi-ye Hanǰan*. (Farhangestān-e zabān va adab-e fārsi. Našr-e āsār 20). Tehrān 1383/2004.

ĀRYĀNPUR KĀŠĀNI 1979 = ĀRYĀNPUR KĀŠĀNI, 'A. – ĀRYĀNPUR KĀŠĀNI, M.: *Farhang-e ǰibi fārsi be englisi*. Tehrān 1358/1979.

ĀSEF FEKRAT 1997 = ĀSEF FEKRAT, M.: *Fārsi-e heravi. Zabān-e goftāri-e Herāt*. (Entešārāt-e Dānešgāh-e Ferdowsi-e Mašhad 215). Mašhad 1376/1997.

ASLANOV 1966 = ASLANOV, M. G.: *Afgansko-russkij slovar' (puštu) : 50000 slov. Pod red. N. A. Dvorjankova*. Moskva 1966.

AŠRAF ALKETĀBI 1983 = AŠRAF ALKETĀBI, M.: 'Farhang-e xānsāri', *Fravahr* 280 (1362/1983), 438–447.

AŠRAFI XĀNSĀRI 2004 = AŠRAFI XĀNSĀRI, M.: *Guyeš-e xānsāri*. (Pežuhešgāh-e ^{c}olum-e ensāni va motālehāt-e farhangi). Tehrān 1383/2004.

AWRANG 1969 = AWRANG, M.: *Farhang-e kordi, «p – t»*. Tehrān 1348/1969.

AYYUBI 2002 = AYYUBI, A.: *Dastur-e zạbān-e fārsi be baluči*. Irānšahr 1381/2002.

ĀZĀDIXĀH 1983 = ĀZĀDIXĀH, M. ^{c}A.: 'Vāžehā-ye ^{c}amiāne va mahalli-e Sirǰān', *Fravahr* 273–274 (1362/1983), 818–822.

AZAMI – WINDFUHR 1972 = AZAMI, Ch. A. – WINDFUHR, G. L.: *A dictionary of Sangesari with a grammatical outline*. Tehran 1972.

BĀBAK 1996 = BĀBAK, ^{c}A.: *Barresi-ye zabānšenāxti. Guyeš-e Zarand*. Kermān 1375/1996.

BĀBĀN 1982 = BĀBĀN, Š.: *Farhang-e fārsi-kordi*. Tehrān 1361/1982.

BADAXŠI 1960 = BADAXŠI, Š. [= Šāh ^{c}Abdullāh]: *Də Afγānistān də cīno žəbo o lahǰo qāmus / Dictionary of some languages and dialects of Afghanistan*. Paṣ̌to Ṭolana [Kābul] 1339/1960.

BAHĀR 1966 = BAHĀR, M.: *Vāženāme-ye Bondaheš*. (Entešārāt-e boniād-e farhang-e Irān 17. Vāženāmehā-ye pahlavi 1). Tehrān 1345/1966.

BAHRĀMI 1990 = BAHRĀMI, E.: *Farhang-e vāžehā-ye avestāi. Bar pāye-ye farhang-e Kangā va negareš be farhanghā-ye digar*. 4 voll. Tehrān 1369/1999.

BAILEY 1933 = BAILEY, H. W. : *The Greater Bundahišn*. Doct. Diss., Oxford University 1933.

BAILEY 1933–1935 = BAILEY, H. W. : 'Iranian studies IV', *Bulletin of the School of Oriental Studies* 7 (1933–1935), 755–778.

BAILEY 1945 = BAILEY, H. W.: 'Asica', *Transactions of the Philological Society* (1945), 1–38.

BAILEY 1954 = BAILEY, H. W.: 'Indo-Iranian studies-II', *Transactions of the Philological Society* (1954), 129–156.

BAILEY 1979 = BAILEY, H. W.: *Dictionary of Khotan Saka*. Cambridge 1979.

BALSAN 1969 = BALSAN, F. : *Étrange Baloutchistan. Photographies et dessins de l'auteur*. (Connaissance de l'Asie). Paris 1969.

BARBERA 2004 BARBERA, G.: *Lingua e cultura a Minâb (Iran sud-orientale). Profilo grammaticale, testi e vocabolario*. PhD diss., Università degli studi di Napoli L'Orientale 2004.

BARKER –MENGAL 1969 = BARKER, M. A. – MENGAL, A. Kh.: *A course in Baluchi*. 2 voll. Montreal 1969.

BARTHOLOMAE 1904 = BARTHOLOMAE, CHR.: *Altiranisches Wörterbuch*. Strassburg 1904.

BARUMAND SA'ID 1991 = BARUMAND SA'ID, J.: *Vāženāme-ye guyeš-e Bardesir*. Tehrān 1370/1991.

BASTAKI 1980 = BASTAKI, ᶜA.A.: *Farhang-e bastaki*. n.p. 1359/1980.

BAU 2003 = BAU, P.: *Dictionnaire persan-français / français-persan*. Paris 2003.

BAZIN 1981 = BAZIN, M.: 'Quelques échantillons des variations dialectales du Tāleši', *Studia Iranica* 10 (1981), 111–281.

BEHRANGI – DEHQĀNI 1348/1969 = BEHRANGI, S. – DEHQĀNI, B.: *Afsānehā-ye Āzerbāiǰān*. Tehrān 1348/1969.

BEHRUZI 1969 = BEHRUZI, ᶜA. N.: *Vāžehā va masalhā-ye širāzi va kāzeruni*. Tehrān 1348/1969.

BEHRUZI 2002 = BEHRUZI, M. J.: *Golhā-ye šahr-e sabz (ešᶜāri be lahǰe-ye mahalli-e kāzeruni)*. (Farhangestān-e zabān va adab-e fārsi. Našr-e āsār 11). Tehrān 1381/2202.

BEHZĀDI 1990 = BEHZĀDI, B.: *Farhang-e āzerbāiǰāni-fārsi*. Tehrān 1369/1990.

BENNETT 1982 = BENNETT, J.: 'The name of the ring-finger in the Germanic languages', *Amsterdamer Beiträge zur älteren Germanistik* 17 (1982), 13–21.

BENVENISTE 1940 = BENVENISTE, E.: *Textes sogdiens édités, traduits et commentés*. (Mission Pelliot en Asie Centrale - Série in-quarto 3). Paris 1940.

BENZING – TARAF 1983 = BENZING, J.: *Chwaresmischer Wortindex, mit einer Einleitung von H. Humbach herausgegeben von Zahra TARAF*. Wiesbaden 1983.

BLANK 2001 = BLANK, A.: 'Words and Concepts in Time : towards Diachronic Cognitive Onomasiology', *Metaphorik.de* 01/2001 [http: // www.metaphorik.de/01/blank.htm].

BLAU 1975 = BLAU, J.: *Le kurde de ᶜAmādiya et de Djabal Sindjār : analyse linguistique, textes folkloriques, glossaries*. (Travaux de l'Institut d'études iraniennes de l'Université de la Sorbonne nouvelle, 8). Paris 1975.

BLAŽEK 2000 = BLAŽEK, V., 'Indo-European "five"', *Indogermanische Forschungen* 105, 101–119

BONFANTE 1939 = BONFANTE, G.: 'Études sur le tabou dans les langues indo-européennes', in *Mélanges de linguistiques offerts à Charles Bally sous les auspices de la Faculté des lettres de l'Université de Genève par des collègues, des confrères, des disciples reconnaissants*. Genève 1939, 195–207.

BONFANTE 1958 = BONFANTE, G.: 'Sull'animismo delle parti del corpo in indoeuropeo', *Ricerche linguistiche* IV (1958), 19–28.

BORĀZJĀNI 2003 = BORĀZJĀNI, T.: *Sir-i dar guyeš-e daštestāni*. Širāz 1382/2003.

BOŠRĀ 2002 = BOŠRĀ, M.: *Han.gi i-sə, han-gi ni-yə. Ketābi dar čistān-e «masalə»-e gilaki*. Rašt 1381/2002.

BOYCE 1954 = BOYCE, M.: *The Manichaean Hymn-Cycles in Parthian*. (London Oriental Series 3). London – New York – Toronto 1954.

BRACCHI 2009 = BRACCHI, R.: *Nomi e volti della paura nelle valli dell'Adda e della Mera*. Tübingen 2009.

BRAY 1934 = BRAY, D.: *The Brāhūī language*. Part II: *The Brāhūī problem*. Part III: *Etymological vocabulary*. Delhi 1934.

BROWN 2005 = BROWN, C.: '130: Finger and hand', in HASPELMATH, M. – DRYER, M. S. – GIL, D. (eds.), *The World Atlas of Language Structures*. Oxford 2005, 526–529.

BROWN – WITKOWSKI 1981 = BROWN, C. H. – WITKOWSKI, S. R.: 'Figurative language in a universalist perspective', *American Ethnologist* 8 (1981), 596–615.

BUCK 1949 = BUCK, C. D.: *A dictionary of selected synonyms in the principal Indo-European languages. A contribution to the history of the ideas*. Chicago 1949 [repr. 1988].

BURNOUF 1845 = BURNOUF, M. E. : 'Études sur la langue et sur les textes zends. IV: Le dieu Homa (suite)', *Journal Asiatique* 1845, 249–308.

BURROW – EMENEAU 1984 = BURROW, T. – EMENEAU, M. B.: *A Dravidian etymological dictionary*. Oxford[2] 1984.

CABOLOV 1976 = CABOLOV, R. L.: *Očerk istoričeskoj fonetiki kurdskogo jazyka*. Moskva 1976.

CABOLOV 2001 = CABOLOV, R. L.: *Ėtimologičeskij slovar' kurdskogo jazyka*. Moskva 2001.

CHANTRAINE 1980 = CHANTRAINE, P. : *Dictionnaire étymologique de la langue grecque. Histoire des mots*. Paris 1980 [2nd ed. 1999].

CHEBEL 1995 = CHEBEL, M. : *Dictionnaire des symboles musulmans. Rites, mystique et civilization*. Paris 1995.

CHEBEL 1999 = CHEBEL, M.: *Le Corps en Islam*. Paris 1999 [first ed. 1984].

CHODŻKO 1842 = CHODŻKO, A.: *Specimens of the popular poetry of Persia as found in the adventures and improvisations of Kurroglou, the bandit-minstrel of Northern Persia and in the songs of the people inhabiting the shores of the Caspian Sea, orally collected and translated with philological and historical notes by A. Chodzko*. London 1842 [repr. New York 1971].

CHEUNG 2005 = CHEUNG, J.: Review of MORGENSTIERNE 2003, *Bulletin of the School of Oriental and African Studies* 68 (2005), 127–129.

CHEUNG 2007 = CHEUNG, J. : *Etymological dictionary of the Iranian verb*. (Leiden Indo-European Etymological Dictionary Series 2). Leiden – Boston 2007.

CHRISTENSEN 1930 = CHRISTENSEN, A.: *Contribution à la dialectologie iranienne* I. *Dialecte guiläki de Recht, dialectes de Färizänd, de Yaran et de Natanz.*

(Det Kgl. Danske Videnskabernes Selskab. Historisk-filologiske Meddelelser XVII, 2). København 1930.

CHRISTENSEN – BARR 1939 = CHRISTENSEN, A.: *Iranische Dialektaufzeichnungen aus dem Nachlaß von F. C. Andreas. Zusammen mit K. Barr und W. Henning bearbeitet und herausgegeben von A. Christensen. Erster Teil:. Sîvändî, Yäzdî und Sôî, bearbeitet von A. Christensen. Kurdische Dialekte, bearbeitet von Kaj Barr.* (Abhandlungen der Gesellschaft der Wissenschaften zu Göttingen. Philologisch-historische Klasse III, 11). Berlin 1939.

CHYET 2003 = CHYET, M. L.: *Kurdish-English dictionary / Ferhenga Kurmancî-Inglîzî.* (Yale Language Series). Yale 2003.

CIPRIANO 1998 = CIPRIANO, P.: *La labiovelare iranica. Dalle sue origini indoeuropee agli sviluppi attuali.* (Biblioteca di ricerche linguistiche e filologiche 48).Viterbo – Roma 1998.

COLETTI 1981 = COLETTI, A.: *Baluchi of Mirjave (Iran). Liku couplets.* Roma 1981.

COLLETT 1983 = COLLETT, N. A.: *A grammar, phrase book and vocabulary of Baluchi* (*as spoken in the Sultanate of Oman*). Abingdon 1983.

CREVATIN 1978 = CREVATIN, F.: 'Due problemi di storia linguistica aria', *Incontri linguistici* 4 (1978), 7-30.

DĀDMĀN 1976 = DĀDMĀN, N.: *Dastur-e zabān va tatavvor va farhang-e lahǰe-ye Esfāhān.* Esfāhān 1355/1976.

DAMES 1891 = DAMES, M. L.: *A text book of the Balochi language, consisting of miscellaneous stories, legends, poems and a Balochi-English vocabulary.* Lahore 1891.

DĀNEŠGAR 1995 = DĀNEŠGAR, A.: *Farhang-e vāžehā-ye rāyeǰ-e Turbat Haydarie.* Mašhad 1374/1995.

DARMESTETER 1880 = DARMESTETER, J.: *The Zend-Avesta.* Part I. *The Vendîdâd.* (The Sacred Book of the East 4). Oxford 1880.

DARMESTETER 1883 = DARMESTETER, J.: *The Zend-Avesta.* Part II. *The Sîrôzahs, Yasts and Nyâyis.* (The Sacred Book of the East 23). Oxford 1883.

DARUDIĀN 1986 = DARUDIĀN, V.: 'Guyeš-e Naqusān', *Farhang-e Irānzamin* 26 (1365/1986), 78–108.

DARVIŠIĀN 1996 = DARVIŠIĀN, ᶜA. A.: *Farhang-e kordi-e kermānšāhi: kordi-fārsi.* Tehrān 1375/1996.

DE CHIARA 2008 = DE CHIARA, M.: *Studi sul lessico e sulla fonetica della lingua pashto.* PhD thesis. Università degli Studi di Napoli "L'Orientale" 2008.

DEETERS – KNOBLOCH 1981 = DEETERS, G. – KNOBLOCH, J.: 'Ein südossetischer Text (Aul wachtᶜānam)', in *Monumentum Morgenstierne* I. (Acta Iranica 21. Deuxième série. Hommages et opera minora VII). Leiden 1981, 99–102.

DEGENER 1989 = DEGENER, A.: *Khotanische Suffixe.* (Alt- und neu-indische Studien 39). Stuttgart 1989.

DEHGHAN 1970 = DEHGHAN, I.: 'The Persian dialect of Āvarzamān', *Journal of Near Eastern Studies* 29 (1970), 259–272.

DEHQĀNI 1998 = DEHQĀNI, E. N.: *Barresi-ye guyeš-e Jiroft va Kahnuǰ.* Kermān 1377/1998.

DEHXODĀ 1946-1981 = DEHXODĀ, A. A.: *Loγātnāme*. Tehrān 1325/1946 – 1360/1981.

DEYHIM 2005 = DEYHIM, G.: *Barresi-e xorde-ye guyešhā-ye mantaqe-ye Qasrān be enzemām-e vāženāme-ye qasrāni*. (Farhangestān-e zabān va adab-e fārsi. Našr-e āsār 88). Tehrān 1384/2005.

DOERFER 1967 = DOERFER, G.: *Türkische Lehnwörter im Tadschikischen*. (Abhandlungen für die Kunde des Morgenlandes 37, 3). Wiesbaden 1967.

DOERFER – HESCHE 1993 = DOERFER, G. – HESCHE, W.: *Chorasantürkisch: Wörterlisten, Kurzgrammatiken, Indices*. (Turcologica 16). Wiesbaden 1993.

DULLING 1973 = DULLING, G. K.: *The Hazaragi Dialect of Afghan Persian: a preliminary study*. (Central Asian Monograph 1). London 1973.

DURKIN-MEISTERERNST 2004 = DURKIN-MEISTERERNST, D.: *Dictionary of Manichaean Middle Persian and Parthian*. (Corpus Fontium Manichaeorum. Dictionary of Manichaean Texts III. Texts from Central Asia and China, part 1). Turnhout 2004.

EBELING 1957 = EBELING, E.: 'Finger', in *Reallexikon der Assyriologie*, 3. Leipzig – Berlin 1957, 66.

EBRĀHIMPUR 1994a = EBRĀHIMPUR, M. T.: *Vāženāme-ye kordi-fārsi*. Tehrān 1373/1994.

EBRĀHIMPUR 1994b = EBRĀHIMPUR, M. T.: *Vāženāme-ye fārsi-kordi*. Tehrān 1373/1994.

ĖDEL'MAN 1971 = ĖDEL'MAN, D. I.: *Yazguljamsko-russkij slovar'*. Moskva 1971.

EDELMAN 1999 = EDELMAN, D. I.: 'On the history of non-decimal systems and their elements in numerals of Aryan languages', in GVOZDANOVIĆ, J. (ed.), *Numeral types and changes worldwide*. (Trends in linguistics. Studies and monographs 118). Berlin 1999, 221-242.

EILERS 1957 = EILERS, W.: 'Akkad. *kaspum* „Silber, Geld“ und Sinnverwandtes', *Welt des Orients* 2/4 (1957), 322–337.

EILERS 1970 = EILERS, W.: 'Die Namen der Kuschan-Könige', in TILAKASIRI, J. (ed.), *Añjali; papers on Indology and Buddhism, a felicitation volume presented to Oliver Hector de Alwis Wijesekera on his sixties birthday*. University of Ceylon 1970, 112–127.

EILERS 1974 = EILERS, W.: 'Herd und Feuerstätte in Iran', in MAYRHOFER, M. (ed.), *Antiquitates Indogermanicae. Studien zur indogermanischen Altertumskunde und zur Sprach- und Kulturgeschichte der indogermanischen Völker. Gedenkschrift für Hermann Güntert fur 25. Wiederkehr seines Todestages am 23. April 1973*. (Innsbrucker Beiträge zur Sprachwissenschaft 12). Innsbruck 1974, 307–338.

EILERS 1976 = EILERS, W.: *Die Mundart von Chunsar*. [...] *Unter Mitarbeit von Ulrich SCHAPKA*. (Westiranische Mundarten aus der Sammlung Wilhelm Eilers I). Wiesbaden 1976.

EILERS 1979 = EILERS, W.: *Die Mundart von Gäz*. [...] *Unter Mitarbeit von Ulrich SCHAPKA*. (Westiranische Mundarten aus der Sammlung Wilhelm Eilers II). 2 voll. Wiesbaden 1979.

EILERS 1988 = EILERS, W.: *Die Mundart von Sīvänd*. (Westiranische Mundarten aus der Sammlung Wilhelm Eilers III). Stuttgart 1988.

EILERS 1990 = EILERS, W.: 'Kūhpāye, das alte Vīr, und seine Mundart', *Bulletin of the Asia Institute* 4 (1990), 217–229.

ELFENBEIN 1963 = ELFENBEIN, J.: *A vocabulary of Marw Baluchi.* (Istituto Universitario Orientale di Napoli. Quaderni della sezione linguistica degli Annali 2). Naples 1963.

ELFENBEIN 1967 = ELFENBEIN, J.: "Laṇḍa, Zor Wəla! Waṇecī", *Archiv Orientální* 35 (1967), 563–606.

ELFENBEIN 1983a = ELFENBEIN, J.: *A Baluchi Miscellanea of Erotica and Poetry: Codex Oriental Additional 24048 of the British Library*, Suppl. n. 35 agli Annali dell'Istituto Universitario Orientale di Napoli 43 (1983), fasc. 2. Napoli 1983.

ELFENBEIN 1983b = ELFENBEIN, J.: 'A Brahui supplementary vocabulary', *Indo-Iranian Journal* 25 (1983), 191–209.

ELFENBEIN 1984 = ELFENBEIN, J. H.: 'The Wanetsi Connection, Part II: Glossary', *Journal of the Royal Asiatic Society* 1984, 229–241.

ELFENBEIN 1990 = ELFENBEIN, J.: *An Anthology of Classical and Modern Balochi Literature.* Vol. I: *Anthology*, Vol. II: *Glossary*. Wiesbaden 1990.

ELFENBEIN 1992 = ELFENBEIN, J.: 'Measurement of time and space in Balochi', *Studia Iranica* 21 (1992), 247–254.

EMĀM 2000 = EMĀM (AHVĀZI), M.: *Čistān-nāme-ye dezfuli.* Moqaddame: *Nazari be adabiāt-e ᶜāmme-ye Irān*, by ᶜA. BOLUKBĀŠI. (Farhang va mardom 4). Tehrān 1379/2000.

EMENEAU – BURROW 1962 = EMENEAU, M. B. – BURROW, T.: *Dravidian borrowings from Indo-Aryan.* (University of California Publications in Linguistics 26). Berkeley – Los Angeles 1962.

EMMERICK 1968 = EMMERICK, R. E.: *Saka grammatical studies.* (London Oriental Series 20). London 1968.

EMMERICK 1982 = EMMERICK, R. E.: '*ttīla* 'tree, shrub'', in EMMERICK, R. E. – SKJÆRVØ, P. O., *Studies in the vocabulary of Khotanese* I. (Sitzungsberichte der Österreichischen Akademie der Wissenschaften. Philosophisch-historische Klasse, 401 / Veröffentlichungen der Iranischen Kommission 12). Wien 1982, 51.

EMMERICK 1993 = EMMERICK, R. E.: '"Boys" and "Girls" in Khotanese', *Bulletin of the Asia Institute*, N.S. 7 (1993), 51–54 [= *Iranian studies in Honor of A. D. Bivar*, ed. by C. A. BROMBERG].

EQTEDĀRI 1951 = EQTEDĀRI, A.: 'Masalhā-ye lārestāni', *Farhang-e Irānzamin*, 30/2 (1330/1951), 233–253.

EQTEDĀRI 1955 = EQTEDĀRI, A.: *Farhang-e lārestāni.* Tehrān 1334/1955.

EQTEDĀRI 1963 = EQTEDĀRI, A.: 'Lahǰe-ye fišarvi', *Farhang-e Irānzamin* 11 (1342/1963), 71–91.

ERDAL 1981 = ERDAL, M.: 'Les doigts coupables des Turcs', in DE SIVERS 1981, 121–126.

FARAHVAŠI 1976 = FARAHVAŠI, B.: *Vāženāme-ye xuri.* (Entešārāt-e vezārat-e farhang va honar. Markaz-e mardomšenāsi-ye Irān 12). Tehrān 2535/1976.

FARĀMARZI 1984 = FARĀMARZI, H.: *Farhang-e Farāmarzān.* Tehrān 1363/1984.

FARHÂDI 1955 = FARHÂDI, A.: *Le persan parlé en Afghanistan. Grammaire du Kâboli, accompagnée d'un recueil de quatrains populaires de la région de Kâbol.* Paris 1955.

FARISOV 1957 = FARISOV, I. O. : *Russko-kurdskij slovar'*. Moskva 1957.

FARZPUR MĀČIĀNI 1954–1955 = FARZPUR MĀČIĀNI, M. : 'Zabān va farhang-e Māčiān', *Našrie-ye Dāneškade-ye adabiāt-e Tabriz* 16/3 (1343/1954), 277–296, 16/4, 451–470; 17/1 (1344/1955), 109–128; 17/2, 261–284.

FATTAH 2000 = FATTAH, I. K.: *Les dialectes kurdes méridionaux. Étude linguistique et dialectologique*. (Acta Iranica 37). Lovanii 2000.

FĀZELI 2004 = FĀZELI, M. T.: *Farhang-e guyeš-e šuštari. Rišešenāsi va moqāyese bā fārsi va guyešhā-ye irāni. Zarb-o-masalhā, nemunehā, vāženāme*. Tehrān 1383/2004.

FILIPPONE 1995 = FILIPPONE, E.: *The "pupil of the eye" in the Iranian languages*. (Etnolinguistica dell'area iranica 5). Napoli 1995.

FILIPPONE 1996 = FILIPPONE, E.: *Spatial models and locative expressions in Baluchi*. (Baluchistan Monograph Series IV). Naples 1996.

FILIPPONE 2000–2003 = FILIPPONE, E.: 'The fingers' names in Balochi', *Balochistan Studies*, 8–10 (2000–2003), 59–89.

FILIPPONE 2006 = FILIPPONE, E.: 'The Body and the landscape. Metaphorical strategies in the lexicon of the Iranian languages', in PANAINO, A. – ZIPOLI, R. (eds.), *Proceedings of the 5th Conference of the Societas Iranologica Europœa held in Ravenna, 6–11 October 2003*. Vol. II. *Classical & contemporary Iranian studies*. Milano 2006, 365–389.

FLEURIOT 1981 = FLEURIOT, L.: 'La main et les doigts dans les langues celtiques', in DE SIVERS 1981, 135–139.

FOWLER – FOWLER 1919 = FOWLER, H. W. – FOWLER, F. G., *The Concise Oxford Dictionary of Current English*. Adapted by H. W. FOWLER and F. G. FOWLER, authors of 'The King's English' from *The Oxford Dictionary*. Oxford 1919.

FRYE 1949 = FRYE, R.N.: 'Report on a trip to Iran in the summer of 1948', *Oriens* 2 (1949), 204–215.

GARUSIN 1991 = GARUSIN, H.: *Vāženāme-ye hamadāni*. Hamadān 1370/1991.

GAUTHIOT 1916 = GAUTHIOT, M. R.: 'Notes sur le yazgoulami, dialecte iranien des confins du Pamir', *Journal Asiatique* (1916), 239–270.

GEIGER 1890–1891 = GEIGER, W.: *Etymologie des Balūčī*. (Abhandlungen der königlichen bayerischen Akademie der Wissenschaften. Philosophisch-philologische Classe, 19,1). München 1890–1891.

GERSHEVITCH 1959 = GERSHEVITCH, I.: *The Avestan Hymn to Mithra. With an introduction, translation and commentary*. (University of Cambridge – Oriental Publication 4). Cambridge 1959. [repr. 1967].

GERSHEVITCH 1964a = GERSHEVITCH, I.: 'Iranian chronological adverbs', in *Indo-Iranica. Mélanges présentés à Georg Morgenstierne, à l'occasion de son soixante-dixième anniversaire*. Wiesbaden 1964, 78–88.

GERSHEVITCH 1964b = GERSHEVITCH, I.: 'Dialect Variation in early Persian', *Transactions of the Philological Society* 1964 [1965], 1–29.

GERSHEVITCH 1996 = GERSHEVITCH, I.: 'A helping hand from Central Asia', in *Convegno Internazionale sul Tema La Persia e l'Asia Centrale da Alessandro al X secolo. (Roma, 9–12 novembre 1994)*. (Atti dei Convegni Lincei 127). Roma 1996, 49–75.

GHARIB 1995 = GHARIB, B.: *Sogdian Dictionary. Sogdian-Persian-English.* Tehrān 1995.

GIGNOUX 1984 = GIGNOUX, Ph.: *Le livre d'Ardā Vīrāz. Transliteration, transcription et traduction du texte pehlevi.* (Bibliothèque iranienne 30 – Cahier 14). Paris 1984.

GIGNOUX – TAFAZZOLI 1993 = GIGNOUX, Ph. – TAFAZZOLI, A., *Anthologie de Zādspram: édition critique du texte pehlevi.* (Studia Iranica – Cahier 13). Paris 1993.

GILBERTSON 1925 = GILBERTSON, G. W.: *English-Balochí colloquial dictionary.* Hertford 1925.

GILBERTSON 1932 = GILBERTSON, G. W.: *The Pakkhto idiom. A dictionary.* By [...] assisted by Árif Ullah Yúsufzai, Mahmúd Afrídí, Alí Akbar Khán Qandahárí. 2 voll. Hertford 1932.

GIPPERT 2009 = GIPPERT, J.: 'An etymological trifle', in SUNDERMANN, W. – HINTZE, A. – DE BLOIS, F. (eds.), *Exegisti monumenta. Festschrift in honour of Nicholas Sims-Williams.* (Iranica 17). Wiesbaden 2009, 127–140.

GNERRE 1995 = GNERRE, M.: 'All'origine dei numerali: conteggiando la numeralità', in *Atti del Convegno su «Numeri e istanze di numerazione tra preistoria e protostoria linguistica del mondo antico» (Napoli, 1–2 dicembre 1995). = AIΩN. Annali del Dipartimento del Mondo Classico e del Mediterraneo Antico – Sezione linguistica* 17 (1995), 121–159.

GOODELL 1979 = GOODELL, G.: 'Bird lore in Southwestern Iran', *Asian Folklore Studies* 32/2 (1979), 131–153.

GRIERSON 1921 = GRIERSON, G. A.: *Specimens of languages of the Eranian family.* (Linguistic Survey of India 10). Calcutta 1921.

GRONDELAERS – GEERAERTS 2003 = GRONDELAERS, S. – GEERAERTS, D.: 'Towards a pragmatic model of cognitive onomasiology', in CUICKENS, H. – DIRVEN, R. – TAYLOR, J. R., *Cognitive approaches to lexical semantics.* Berlin – New York 2003, 67–92.

GRJUNBERG 1963 = GRJUNBERG , A. L.: *Jazyk severoazerbajdžanskix tatov.* Leningrad 1963.

GRJUNBERG 1972 = GRJUNBERG, A. L.: *Jazyki vostočnogo Gindukuša. Mundžanskij jazyk. Teksty. Slovar'. Grammatičeskij očerk.* Leningrad 1972.

GRJUNBERG – STEBLIN-KAMENSKIJ 1976 = GRJUNBERG, A. L. – STEBLIN-KAMENSKIJ, I. M.: *Jazyki vostočnogo Gindukuša. Vaxanskij jazyk. Teksty, slovar', grammatičeskij očerk.* Moskva 1976.

HADANK 1930 = HADANK, K.: *Mundarten der Gûrân, besonders das Kändûläî, Auramânî und Bâdschälânî.* (Kurdisch-persische Forschungen: Ergebnisse einer von 1901 bis 1903 und 1906 bis 1907 in Persien und der asiatische Türkei ausgeführten Forschungsreise von Oskar Mann. Abt. 3 (Nordwestiranisch), 2). Berlin 1930.

HADANK 1932 = HADANK, K.: *Mundarten der Zâzâ, hauptsächlich aus Siwerek and Kor.* (Kurdisch-persische Forschungen: Ergebnisse einer von 1901 bis 1903 und 1906 bis 1907 in Persien und der asiatische Türkei ausgeführten Forschungsreise von Oskar Mann. Abt. 3 (Nordwestiranisch), 4). Berlin 1932.

HAIM 1992a = HAIM, S.: *Farhang-e bozorg-e fārsi-englisi.* Tehrān 1371/1992.

HAIM 1992b = HAIM, S.: *Farhang-e bozorg-e englisi-fārsi*. Tehrān 1371/1992.

HAKIM 1996 = HAKIM, H.: *Dictionnaire fondamental kurde-français. Dialecte sorani*. (Dictionnaires L&M Langues O'). Paris 1996.

HAKIM – GAUTIER 1993 = HAKIM, H. – GAUTIER, G.: *Dictionnaire français-kurde*. Paris 1993.

HAMIDI 2001 = HAMIDI, J. : *Farhangnāme-ye Bušehr*. Tehrān 1380/2001.

HASURI 1964 = HASURI, ᶜA.: *Gozāreš-e guyešhā-ye lori*. (Zabān va farhang-e Irān 28). Tehrān 1343/1964.

HAŽĀR 1990 = HAŽĀR: *Farhang-e kordi-fārsi*. Tehrān 1369/1990.

HEJĀZI KENĀRI 1995 = HEJĀZI KENĀRI, H.: *Vāženāme-ye māzandarāni va rišehā-ye ānhā*. Tehrān 1374/1995.

HENNING 1937 = HENNING, W. B., 'A list of Middle Persian and Parthian words', *Bulletin of the School of Oriental Studies* 9 (1937), 79–92 [= HENNING 1977, I, 559–572].

HENNING 1939 = HENNING, W. B.: 'Sogdian loan-words in New Persian', *Bulletin of the School of Oriental Studies* 10 (1939), 93–106. [= HENNING 1977, I, 639–652].

HENNING 1942 = HENNING, W. B.: 'An astronomical chapter of the Bundahishn', *Journal of the Royal Asiatic Society* (1942), 229–248. [= HENNING 1977, II, 95–114].

HENNING 1945 = HENNING, W. B.: 'Sogdian tales', *Bulletin of the School of Oriental and African Studies* 11, 3 (1945), 465–487. [= HENNING 1977, II, 169–191].

HENNING 1948 = HENNING, W. B.: 'Oktō(u)', *Transactions of the Philological Society* (1948), 69. [= HENNING 1977, II, 347].

HENNING 1954 = HENNING, W. B.: 'The ancient language of Azerbaijan', *Transactions of the Philological Society* (1954), 157–177. [= HENNING 1977, II, 457–477].

HENNING 1956 = HENNING, W. B.: 'The Khwarezmian language', in *Zeki Velidi Togan'a Armağan / Symbolae in Honorem Z. V. Togan*. Istanbul 1950–1955. Istanbul 1956, 421–436. [= HENNING 1977, II, 485–500].

HENNING 1958 = HENNING, W. B.: 'Mitteliranisch', in SPULER, B. (ed.), *Handbuch der Orientalistik. I, IV, 1. Linguistik*. Leiden – Köln 1958, 20–129.

HENNING 1965 = HENNING, W. B.: 'Surkh Kotal und Kaniṣka', *Zeitschrift der Deutschen Morgenländischen Gesellschaft* (1965), 75–87. [= HENNING 1977, II, 631–643].

HENNING 1977 = HENNING, W. B.: *Selected Papers*, I. (Acta Iranica 14. Deuxième série. Hommages et opera minora V). II. (Acta Iranica 15. Deuxième série. Hommages et opera minora VI). Téhéran-Liège 1977.

HETU RAM 1898 = HETU RAM, R. B.: *Translation of the Bilochi-nama compiled by Rai Bahadur HETU RAM*. (transl. revised by J. McC DOUIE). Lahore 1898.

HINTON – NICHOLS – OHALA 1994 = HINTON, L. – NICHOLS, J. – OHALA, J. (eds.): *Sound symbolism*. Cambridge 1995.

HINTZE 1994 = HINTZE, A.: *Der Zamyād-Yašt. Edition, Übersetzung, Kommentar*. (Beiträge zur Iranistik 15). Wiesbaden 1994.

HOMĀYUN 1992a = HOMĀYUN, S.: *Farhang-e mardom-e Sarvestān*. Tehrān 1371/1992.

HOMĀYUN 1992b = HOMĀYUN, H.: *Guyeš-e aftari*. (Mo'assese-ye motāleᶜāt va tahqiqāt-e farhangi 659). Tehrān 1371/1992.

HOMĀYUN 2004 = HOMĀYUN, H.: *Guyeš-e Kalimiān-e Yazd* (*yek guyeš-e irāni*). Tehrān 1383/2004.

HOPTAM 2000 = HOPTAM, A.: '*Finger* and some other *f-* and *fl-*words', *North-Western European Language Evolution* 36 (2000), 77–91.

HORN 1893 = Horn, P.: *Grundriss der neupersischen Etymologie.* (Sammlung indogermanischer Wörterbücher IV). Strassburg 1893. [repr. 1988].

HORN 1898–1901 = HORN, P.: 'IV. Neupersische Schriftsprache', in GEIGER, W. – KUHN, E., *Grundriss der iranischen Philologie*, I/2. Erster Abschnitt: Sprachgeschichte II. Strassburg 1898–1901, 1–200. [repr. 1974].

HOROWITZ 1992 = HOROWITZ, F. E.: 'On the Proto-Indo-European etymon for 'hand'', *Word* 43/3 (1992), 411–419.

HÜBSCHMANN 1895 = HÜBSCHMANN, H., *Persische Studien.* Strassburg 1895.

HÜBSCHMANN 1897 = HÜBSCHMANN, H., *Armenische Grammatik.* I. Theil. *Armenische Etimologie.* (Bibliothek indogermanischer Grammatiken 6). Leipzig 1897. [repr. 1992].

HUMBACH – ICHAPORIA 1998 = HUMBACH, H. – ICHAPORIA, P. R.: *Zamyād Yasht. Yasht 19 of the Younger Avesta. Text, translation, commentary.* Wiesbaden 1998.

IZADPANĀH 1989 = IZADPANĀH, H.: *Farhang-e lakki.* Tehrān 1368/1989.

IZADPANĀH 2001 = IZADPANĀH, H.: *Farhang-e lori.* (Entešārat-e Asātir 320). Tehrān 1380/2001 [1st ed. 1343/1964].

JABA – JUSTI 1879 = JABA, A.: *Dictionnaire kurde-français,* publié [...] par [...] F. JUSTI. St.-Pétersbourg 1879.

JA^cFARI DEHAQI 2002 = JA^cFARI DEHAQI, M.: 'Guyeš-e Gurkāni', in REZĀI BĀГBIDI, H. (ed.), *Majmu^ce-ye maqālāt-e naxostin hamandiši-e guyeššenāsi-e Irān. 9 tā 11 Ordibehešt. Goruh-e guyeššenāsi.* (Farhangestān-e zabān va adab-e fārsi. Našr-e āsār 24). Tehrān 1381/2002, 143–157.

JAMASP-ASA 1985 = JAMASP-ASA, K. M.: 'On the *Drōn* in Zoroastrianism', in *Papers in honour of Professor Mary Boyce*, I. (Acta Iranica 24. Deuxième série. Hommages et opera minora X). Leiden 1985, 335–356.

JAMASPJI – HAUG 1867 = JAMASPJI, H., *An Old Zand-Pahlavi glossary* (revised with notes and introduction by M. HAUG). Bombay – London 1867.

JUKES 1961 = JUKES, A.: *Dictionary of the Jatki or Western Panjábi language.* Delhi 1961. [1st ed. 1900].

JUSUPOVA 1985 = JUSUPOVA, Z. A.: *Sulejmanijskij dialekt kurdskogo jazyka.* (Jazyki narodov Azii i Afriki). Moskva 1985.

KALAKI 1973 = KALAKI, B.: 'Guyeš-e Baxtiārihā: dehkade-ye Pāgač', *Honar-o-mardom* 134 (1352/1973), 44–47; 64–68.

KALBĀSI 1983 = KALBĀSI, I.: *Guyeš-e kordi-e Mahābād.* (Mo'assese-ye motāle^cāt va tahqiqāt-e farhangi 513). Tehrān 1362/1983.

KALBĀSI 1991 = KALBĀSI, I.: *Fārsi-e Esfahān.* (Mo'assese-ye motāle^cāt va tahqiqāt-e farhangi 648). Tehrān 1370/1991.

KALBĀSI 1994 = KALBĀSI, I.: *Guyeš-e kelimiān-e Esfahān* (*yek guyeš-e irāni*). (Pežuhešgāh-e ^colum-e ensāni va motāle^cāt-e farhangi 762). Tehrān 1373/1994.

KALBĀSI 1995 = KALBĀSI, I.: *Fārsi-e Irān va Tājikestān* (*yek barresi-e moqābelei*). Tehrān 1374/1995.

KALBĀSI 1997 = KALBĀSI, I.: *Guyeš-e Kelārdašt* (*Rudbārak*). (Pežuhešgāh-e ᶜolum-e ensāni va motāleᶜāt-e farhangi). Tehrān 1376/1997.

KAMIOKA – YAMADA 1979 = KAMIOKA, K. – YAMADA, M.: *Lāri basic vocabulary.* (Lārestānī Studies 1). Tokyo 1979.

KAMIOKA – RAHBAR – HAMIDI 1986 = KAMIOKA, K. – RAHBAR, A. – HAMIDI, A. A.: *Comparative basic vocabulary of Khonjī and Lārī.* (Lārestānī Studies 2). Tokyo 1986.

KANGA 1909 = KANGA, K. E.: *English-Avesta dictionary.* Bombay 1909.

KAPADIA 1953 = KAPADIA, D. D.: *Glossary of Pahlavi Vendidad.* Bombay 1953.

KARAMŠOEV 1988 – 1991 – 1999 = KARAMŠOEV, D.: *Šugnansko-russkij slovar'.* Moskva. I, 1988. II, 1991. III, 1999.

KARBĀSI RĀVARI 1987 = KARBĀSI RĀVARI, ᶜA.: *Farhang-e mardom-e Rāvar.* (Boniād-e Nišābur 17). Tehrān 1366.

KĀRENG 1954 = KĀRENG, ᶜA.: *Tāti va Harzani. Do lahǰe az zabān-e bāstān-e Āzerbāiǰān.* Tabriz 1333/1954.

KELLENS 1989 = KELLENS, J.: 'Avestique', in SCHMITT 1989, 32–55.

KIEFFER 1979–1980 = KIEFFER, Ch. M.: 'Études parāči. IVa. Le Lexique parāči: Glossaire', *Studia Iranica* 8/1 (1979), 67–106; 'Études parāči. IVb. Le Lexique parāči: Glossaire', *Studia Iranica* 8/2 (1979), 245–267; 'Études parāči. IVc. Le Lexique parāči: Glossaire', *Studia Iranica* 9/1 (1980), 99–119; 'Études parāči. IVd. Le Lexique parāči: Glossaire', *Studia Iranica* 9/2 (1980), 233–306.

KLINGENSCHMITT 1968 = KLINGENSCHMITT, G.: *Farhang-i ōīm. Edition und Kommentar*, Inaugural-Dissertation der Philosophischen Fakultät der Friedrich-Alexander-Universität zu Erlangen-Nürnberg 1968 (unpubl.).

KORN 2005 = KORN, A.: *Towards a Historical Grammar of Balochi. Studies in Balochi Historical Phonology and Vocabulary.* (Beiträge zur Iranistik 26). Wiesbaden 2005.

KOTWAL 1969 = KOTWAL, M. P. F.: *The Supplementary texts to the Šāyest nē-šāyest.* København 1969.

KOTWAL – KREYENBROEK 1995 = KOTWAL, F. M. – KREYENBROEK, Ph. G.: *The Hērbedestān and Nērangestān. Volume II. Nērangestān, Fragard 1*, edited and translated by Firoze M. KOTWAL and Philip G. KREYENBROEK with contributions by J. R. RUSSELL. (Studia Iranica – Cahier 16). Paris 1995.

KRAHNKE 1976 = KRAHNKE, K. J.: *Linguistic relationships in Central Iran*, PhD thesis University of Michigan 1976.

KUMAMOTO 1987a = KUMAMOTO, H.: 'tcaṃgalai 'his elbows'', in EMMERICK, R. E. – SKJÆRVØ, P. O., *Studies in the Vocabulary of Khotanese II.* (Sitzungsberichte der Österreichischen Akademie der Wissenschaften. Philosophisch-historische Klasse, 458 / Veröffentlichungen der Iranischen Kommission 17). Wien 1987, 48–49.

KUMAMOTO 1987b = KUMAMOTO, H.: '*hagaiṣṭa 'information'', in EMMERICK, R. E. – SKJÆRVØ, P. O., *Studies in the Vocabulary of Khotanese II.* (Sitzungsberichte der Österreichischen Akademie der Wissenschaften. Philosophisch-historische Klasse, 458 / Veröffentlichungen der Iranischen Kommission 17). Wien 1987, 151–154.

KURDOEV 1957 = KURDOEV, K. K.: *Grammatika kurdskogo jazyka (kurmandži)*. Moskva – Leningrad 1957.

KURDOEV 1960 = KURDOEV, K. K.: *Kurdsko-russkij slovar'*. Moskva 1960.

KURDOEV – JUSUPOVA 1983 = KURDOEV, K. K. – JUSUPOVA, Z.A.: *Kurdsko-russkij slovar' (Sorani)*. Moskva 1983.

LAMBTON 1938 = LAMBTON, A. K. S.: *Three Persian Dialects*. London 1938.

LAMᶜE 1970 = LAMᶜE, M.: *Farhang-e ᶜamiāne-ye ᶜašāyer-e Boyer-Ahmadi va Kuhgiluye*. Tehrān 1349/1970.

LANDI 2000 = LANDI, M.: 'Su una procedura iniziale di computo nell'albanese: mano = cinque', *AIΩN. Annali del Dipartimento di Studi del Mondo Classico e del Mediterraneo Antico – Sezione linguistica* 22 (2000), 185–197.

LANE 1968 = LANE, E. W.: *An Arabic-English Lexicon*. Beirut 1968.

LAZARD 1956 = LAZARD, G.: 'Caractères distinctifs de la langue tadjik', *Bulletin de la Société de Linguistique de Paris* 52 (1956), 117–186.

LAZARD 1963 = LAZARD, G.: *La langue des plus anciens monuments de la prose persane*. (Études linguistiques 2). Paris 1963.

LAZARD 1979 = LAZARD, G.: 'Glossaire Mâsulei', *Studia Iranica* 8 (1979), 269–275.

LAZARD 1990a = LAZARD, G.: *Dictionnaire persan-français*, par [...], avec l'assistance de Mehdi GHAVAM-NEJAD. Leiden/Téhéran 1990.

LAZARD 1990b = LAZARD, G.: 'Le dialect de Rudbār (Gilān)', in *Iranica Varia. Papers in honour of Prof. E. Yarshater*. (Acta Iranica 30. Troisième série. Textes et mémoires XVI). Leiden 1990, 11–23.

LECOQ 1979 = LECOQ, P.: *Le dialect de Sivand*. (Beiträge zur Iranistik 10). Wiesbaden 1979.

LECOQ 1989a = LECOQ, P.: 'Les dialectes caspiens et du nord-ovest', in SCHMITT 1989, 296–312.

LECOQ 1989b = LECOQ, P.: 'Le classement des langues occidentales', in Ph. GIGNOUX – C.-H. de FOUCHÉCOUR, *Études irano-aryennes offertes à Gilbert Lazard*. (Studia Iranica – Cahier 7). Paris 1989, 247–264.

LECOQ 2002 = LECOQ, P.: *Recherches sur les dialectes kermaniens (Iran central). Grammaire, textes, traductions et glossaires*. (Acta Iranica 39). Lovanii 2002.

LENTZ 1933 = LENTZ, W.: *Pamir-Dialekte, I. Materialien zur Kenntnis der Schugni-Gruppe*. (Ergänzungshefte zur Zeitschrift für vergleichende Sprachforschung auf dem Gebiete der indogermanischen Sprachen 12). Göttingen 1933.

LENTZ 1939 = LENTZ, W.: *Zeitrechnung in Nuristan und am Pamir*. (Abhandlungen der Preussischen Akademie der Wissenschaften, Jahrg. 1938, Philosophisch-Historische Klasse 7). Berlin 1939.

LIDDEL – SCOTT 1996 = LIDDEL, H. G. – SCOTT, R.: *A Greek-English Lexicon*. Revised and augmented throughout by Sir H. STUART JONES with the assistence of R. MCKENZIE and with the cooperation of many scholars. With revised supplement. Oxford[9] 1996.

LIRĀVI 2001 = LIRĀVI, A.: *Guyeš va adabiāt-e farhang-e mardom-e Lirāvi va Daylam*. Tehrān 1380/2001.

LORIMER 1922 = LORIMER, D. L. R.: *The Phonology of the Bakhtiari, Badakhshani, and Madaglashti Dialects of Modern Persian, with vocabularies*. (Prize Publication Fund 6). London 1922.

LORIMER 1955 = LORIMER, D. L. R.: 'The popular verse of the Bakhtiāri of S.W. Persia – II. Specimens of Bakhtiāri verse', *Bulletin of the School of Oriental and African Studies* 17 (1955), 93–110.

LORIMER 1958 = LORIMER, D. L. R.: *The Wakhi language 2. Vocabulary and index*. London 1958.

LUCERI 2004 = LUCERI, I. A.: *Dizionario Kurdo-Italiano / Italiano-Kurdo*. Roma 2004

MACKENZIE 1961 = MACKENZIE, D. N.: *Kurdish dialect studies I*. (London Oriental Series 9). London 1961.

MACKENZIE 1966 = MACKENZIE, D. N.: *The dialect of Awroman (Hawrāmān-ī luhōn). Grammatical sketch, texts, and vocabulary*. (Historisk-filosofiske Skrifter udgivet af Det Kongelige Danske Videnskabernes Selskab 4, 3). København 1966.

MACKENZIE 1971 = MACKENZIE, D. N.: *A concise Pahlavi dictionary*. London 1971.

MAGGI 1997a = MAGGI, M.: *Pelliot Chinois 2928. A Khotanese love story*. (Serie Orientale Roma LXXX). Roma 1997.

MAGGI 1997b = MAGGI, M.: 'cäkvaka- 'boy' [not 'as much' as *Dict*. 101b]', in R. E. EMMERICK – P. O. SKJÆRVØ, *Studies in the Vocabulary of Khotanese III*. (Sitzungsberichte der Österreichischen Akademie der Wissenschaften. Philosophisch-historische Klasse, 651 / Veröffentlichungen der Iranischen Kommission 27). Wien 1997, 53–55.

MAHMUDOV 2001 = MAHMUDOV, M.: 'Nazar-i be guyešhā-ye gunāgun-e tājiki', *Noma-i pažūhišgoh / Nāme-ye pežuhešgāh* 1 (2001), 43–47.

MAJIDI 1975 = MAJIDI, M. R.: *Guyešhā-ye pirāmun-e Kāšān va Mahallāt*. (Entešārāt-e Farhangestān-e zabān-e Irān 12). Tehrān 1354/1975.

MALEKZĀDE 2001 =MALEKZĀDE, M. J.: *Farhang-e Zarqān*. (Farhangestān-e zabān va adab-e fārsi. Našr-e āsār 8). Tehrān 1380/2001. (2nd ed.).

MALEKZĀDE 2004 =MALEKZĀDE, M. J.: *Farhang-e masalhā, estelāhāt va kenāyāt-e ᶜāmiāne-ye Zarqān*. Tehrān 1383/2004.

MANN 1909 = MANN, O.: *Die Tâjîk-Mundarten der Provinz Fârs*. (Kurdisch-persische Forschungen 1). Berlin 1909.

MANN 1910 = MANN, O.: *Die Mundarten der Lur-Stämme im südwestlichen Persien*. (Kurdisch-persische Forschungen 2). Berlin 1910.

MARᶜAŠI 2003 = MARᶜAŠI, A.: *Vāženāme-ye guyeš-e gilaki be enzemām-e estelāhāt va zarb-ol-masalhā-ye gilaki*. Rašt 1382/2003. (1st ed. 2535/1976).

MAŠKUR 1978 = MAŠKUR, M. J.: *Farhang-e tatbiqi-e ᶜarabi bā zabānhā-ye sāmi va irāni*. I. (Entešārāt-e bonyād-e farhang-e Irān 276. Zabānšenāsi-e irāni 12). II . (Entešārāt-e bonyād-e farhang-e Irān 277. Zabānšenāsi-e irāni 13). Tehrān 1357/1958.

MAYER 1910 = MAYER, T. J. L.: *English-Biluchi dictionary*. Calcutta 1910.

MAYRHOFER 1979 = MAYRHOFER, M.: *Iranisches Personennamenbuch I. Die altiranischen Namen*. (Sonderpublikation der Iranischen Kommission / Österreichische Akademie der Wissenschaften. Philosophisch-Historische Klasse). Wien 1979.

MAZDĀPUR 1990 = MAZDĀPUR, K.: *Šāyest nāšāyest. Matni be zabān-e pārsi-e miāne. (Pahlavi-e sāsāni)*. (Mo'assese-ye motāle^{c}āt va tahqiqāt-e farhangi 620). Tehrān 1990/1369.

MAZDĀPUR 1995 = MAZDĀPUR, K: *Vāženāme-ye guyeš-e Behdinān-e šahr-e Yazd. Fārsi be guyeš bā mesāl. Jeld-e avval (ā – p)*. (Pežuhešgāh-e ^{c}olum-e ensāni va motāle^{c}āt-e farhangi). Tehrān 1374/1995.

MAZRA^{c}TI *et al.* 1995 = MAZRA^{c}TI, ^{c}A. – MAZRA^{c}TI, ^{c}A. – MAZRA^{c}TI, M.: *Farhang-e bizovoi (Abuzeyd Ābād-e Kāšān)*. Tehrān 1374/1995.

MILITAREV – KOGAN 2000 = MILITAREV, A. – KOGAN, L.: *Semitic Etymological Dictionary*. Vol. I. *Anatomy of Man and Animals*. (Alter Orient und Altes Testament 278). Münster 2000.

MILLER 1930 = MILLER, B. V.: *Talyškie teksty. Teksty, russkij perevod i talyšsko-russko-francuzskij slovar'*. Moskva 1930.

MILLS 1887 = MILLS, L. H.: *The Zend-Avesta*. Part III: *The Yasna, Visparad, Âfrînagân, Gâhs, and miscellanous fragments*. Translated by L. H. MILLS. (The Sacred Books of the East 31). Oxford 1887. [repr. Delhi 1994]

MIRZOZODA 2008 = MIRZOZODA, S.: *Farhang-i yaγnobī-tojikī-anglisī / Yagnob-Tajik-English dictionary*. Dušanbe 2008.

MIRZOZODA – QOSIMI 1995 = MIRZOZODA, S. – QOSIMI, M.: *Farhang-i zabon-i yaγnobi*. Dušanbe 1374/1995.

MIṬHĀ – SURAT 1970 = MIṬHĀ XĀN MARRI – SURAT XĀN: *Baločī-Urdū Luγāt*. Koeṭṭa 1970.

MOHAMMADI XOMAK 2000 = MOHAMMADI XOMAK, J. (SAKĀI-E SISTĀNI): *Vāženāme-ye sakzi (Farhang-e loγāt-e sistāni)*. Tehrān 1379/2000.

MOHTĀT n.d. = MOHTĀT, M. R.: *Simā-ye šahr-e Arāk. Jāme^{c}ešenāsi-ye šahri*. N.p. n.d.

MO^{c}IN 1992 = MO^{c}IN, M.: *Farhang-e fārsi (motavasset)*. 6 voll. Tehrān 1371/1992. (8th ed.).

MOINFAR 1981 = MOINFAR, M. DJ.: 'La main et les doigts dans l'expression linguistique en persan', in DE SIVERS 1981, 223–231.

MOKRI 1966 = MOKRI, M.: *La légende de Bīžan u Manīǰa, version populaire du Sud du Kurdistan en langue gouranie (Épisode du Shahnama, épopée iranienne)*. (Textes et études religieux, linguistiques et ethnographiques. Langue et civilization iraniennes 1). Paris 1966.

MOKRI 2005 = MOKRI, M.: 'Esthétique et lexique du corps humain dans la littérature classique iranienne', *Journal Asiatique* 293/1 (2005), 245–356.

MOLÉ 1993 = MOLÉ, M.: *La légende de Zoroastre selon les texts pehlevis*. (Travaux de l'Institut d'Études Iraniennes de l'Université de Paris 3). Paris 1993 (first ed. 1967).

MONCHI-ZADEH 1990 = MONCHI-ZADEH, D.: *Wörter aus Xurāsān und ihre Herkunft*. (Acta Iranica 29. Troisième série. Textes et mémoires XV). Leiden 1990.

MONIER-WILLIAMS 1899 = MONIER-WILLIAMS, M.: *A Sanskrit-English dictionary etymologically and philologically arranged with special reference to cognate Indo-European languages* [...] with the collaboration of E. LEUMANN, C. CAPPELLER and other scholars. Oxford 1899.

MONTEIL 1954 = MONTEIL, V.: *Le persan contemporain. Textes et vocabulaires*. Paris 1954.

MOQDAM 1949 = MOQDAM, M. : *Guyešhā-ye Vafs o Āštiān o Tafreš*. (Irān Kude 11). Tehrān 1318/1949.

MORANO 2005 = MORANO, E.: 'Preparing the corpus of the Sogdian texts for the SOAS *Manichaean Dictionar Project*', in CERETI, C. G. – MAGGI, M. (eds.), *Middle Iranian Lexicography. Proceedings of the Conference held in Rome, 9–11 April 2001*. (Serie Orientale Roma XCVIII). Roma 2005, 215–223.

MORGENSTIERNE 1927 = MORGENSTIERNE, G.: *An etymological vocabulary of Pashto*. (Skrifter utgitt av det Norske Videnskaps-Akademi i Oslo II, Historisk-filosofisk Klasse 1927, 3). Oslo 1929.

MORGENSTIERNE 1929 = MORGENSTIERNE, G.: *Indo-Iranian frontier languages. Iranian Parachi and Ormuri*. (Instituttet for sammenlignende kulturforksning. Serie B: Skrifter XI). Oslo 1927.

MORGENSTIERNE 1930 = MORGENSTIERNE, G.: 'The Waṇetsi dialect of Pashto', *Norsk Tidsskrift for Sprogvidenskab* 4 (1930), 156–175.

MORGENSTIERNE 1932a = MORGENSTIERNE, G.: 'Notes on Balochi etymology', *Norsk Tidsskrift for Sprogvidenskab* 5 (1932), 37–53.

MORGENSTIERNE 1932b = MORGENSTIERNE, G.: 'Supplementary notes on Ormuri', *Norsk Tidsskrift for Sprogvidenskab* 5 (1932), 5–36.

MORGENSTIERNE 1937 = MORGENSTIERNE, G.: Review of D. BRAY, *The Brāhūī language* II, III, *Journal of the Royal Asiatique Society* (1937), 345–348.

MORGENSTIERNE 1938 = MORGENSTIERNE, G.: *Indo-Iranian frontier languages,* II. *Iranian Pamir languages (Yidgha-Munji, Sanglechi-Ishkashmi and Wakhi)*. (Instituttet for sammenlignende kulturforksning. Serie B: Skrifter XXXV). Oslo 1938.

MORGENSTIERNE 1960 = MORGENSTIERNE, G.: 'Stray notes on Persian dialects', *Norsk Tidsskrift for Sprogvidenskab* 19, (1960) 73–140.

MORGENSTIERNE 1966 = MORGENSTIERNE, G.: 'Notes on the Pashto Ṭolana Vocabulary of Munji', in ASMUSSEN, J. P. – LÆSSØE, J. (eds.), *Iranian studies*. Copenhagen 1966, 177–188.

MORGENSTIERNE 1974 = MORGENSTIERNE, G.: *Etymological vocabulary of the Shughni group*. Wiesbaden 1974.

MORGENSTIERNE 2003 = MORGENSTIERNE, G.: *A new etymological vocabulary of Pashto*. Compiled and edited by J. ELFENBEIN, D. N. MACKENZIE and N. SIMS-WILLIAMS. (Beiträge zur Iranistik 23). Wiesbaden 2003.

MOSALMĀNIĀN QOBĀDIĀNI 1997 = MOSALMĀNIĀN QOBĀDIĀNI, R.: *Zabān va adab-e fārsi dar Farārud*. Tehrān 1376/1997.

MOTAᶜMEDI 2001 = MOTAᶜMEDI, ᶜA.: *Rudān, behešt-e ǰanub*. Bandar ᶜAbbās 1380/2001.

NAGUMAN n.d. = *English-Urdu-Balochi dictionary Naguman*. Unpubl. ms. n.d.

NAJAFI 1999 = NAJAFI, A.: *Farhang-e fārsi-e ᶜāmiāne*. 2 voll. Tehrān 1378/1999.

NAJAFZĀDE-YE BĀRFORUŠ 1989 = NAJAFZĀDE-YE BĀRFORUŠ, M. B.: *Vāženāme-ye māzandarāni*. (Entešārāt-e Boniād-e Nišābur 21). Tehrān 1368/1989.

NAJIBI FINI 2002 = NAJIBI FINI, B.: *Barresi-e guyeš-e fini*. (Farhangestān-e zabān va adab-e fārsi. Našr-e āsār 26). Tehrān 1381/2002.

NAVĀBI 1992 = NAVĀBI, Y. M.: 'Zabān-e konuni-e Āzerbāiǰān', in AFŠĀR, I. (ed.), *Zabān-e fārsi dar Āzerbāiǰān II. Az neveštehā-ye dānešmandān va zabānšenāsān*. Tehrān 1371/1992, 27–178. (first publ. in *Našrie-ye Dāneškade-ye Adabiāt-e Dānešgāh-e Tabriz* 1332/1353).

NAWATA 1982 = NAWATA, T.: 'The Masal dialect of Talishi', in *Monumentum Georg Morgenstierne* II. (Acta Iranica 22, Deuxième série. Hommages et opera minora VIII). Leiden 1982, 93–117.

NIRUMAND 1976 = NIRUMAND, M. B.: *Vāženāme az guyeš-e šuštari*. (Entešārāt-e Farhangestān-e zabān-e Irān 21). Tehrān 2535/1976.

NURBAXŠ 1990 = NURBAXŠ, H.: *Jazire-ye Qešm va xaliǰ-e Fārs*. Tehrān 1369/1990.

NYBERG 1931 = NYBERG, H. S.: *Hilfsbuch des Pehlevi*. II. *Glossar*. Uppsala 1931.

NYBERG 1974 = NYBERG, H. S.: *A manual of Pahlavi*. II. *Ideograms, glossary, abbreviations, index, grammatical survey, corrigenda to Part 1*. Wiesbaden 1974.

OMAR 1992 = OMAR, F. F.: *Kurdisch-Deutsches Wörterbuch (Kurmancî)*. Berlin 1992.

ONIANS 1998 = ONIANS, R. B.: *Le origini del pensiero europeo intorno al corpo, la mente, l'anima, il tempo e il destino*. Milano 1998. [It. transl. from the original: *The origins of European thought about the body, the mind, the soul, the world, time and fate. New interpretations of Greek, Roman and kindred evidence, also of some basic Jewish and Christian beliefs*. Cambridge 1988].

ORANSKIJ 1970 = ORANSKIJ, I. M.: 'K imeni baktrijskogo (?) voždja Κατάνης (IV v. do n. ė.)', *Palestinskij sbornik* 21 [84] (1970), 155–170.

ORANSKIJ 1983 = ORANSKIJ, I. M.: *Tadžikojazyčnye ėtnografičeskie gruppy gissarskoj doliny (Srednjaja Azija). Ėtnolingvističeskoe issledovanie*. Moskva 1983.

ORYĀN 1998 = ORYĀN, S.: *Vāženāme-ye pahlavi-pāzand (Farhang-e pahlavi)*. (Pežuhešgāh-e farhang va honar-e eslāmi. Zabān va adabiāt 4). Tehrān 1377/1998.

PARMĀNAND MĒWĀRĀM 1910 = PARMĀNAND MĒWĀRĀM: *Sindhī-ingliš ḍikšanarī / Sindhi-English Dictionary*. Hyderabad 1910 [repr. 1976].

PARTAVI ĀMOLI 1979 = PARTAVI ĀMOLI, M.: *Farhang-e ᶜavām-e Āmol*. (Vezārat-e farhang va āmuzeš-e ᶜāli. Markaz-e mardomšenāsi-ye Irān 19). Tehrān 1358/1979.

PAUL 1998 = PAUL, L.: *Zazaki. Grammatik und Versuch einer Dialektologie*. (Beiträge zur Iranistik 18). Wiesbaden 1998.

PAXALINA 1959 = PAXALINA, T. N.: *Iškašimskij jazyk. Očerk fonetiki i grammatiki, teksty i slovar'*. Moskva 1959.

PAXALINA 1971 = PAXALINA, T. N.: *Sarykol'sko-russkij slovar'*. Moskva 1971.

PĀYANDE 1987 = PĀYANDE, M. (LANGARUDI): *Farhang-e Gil-o-Deylam. Fārsi be gilaki*. Tehrān 1366/1987.

PIERCE 1875 = PIERCE, E.: 'A description of the Mekranee-Belochee dialect', *Journal of the Bengal Branch of the Royal Asiatic Society* 31, 11 (1875), 1–98.

PIREJKO 1976 = PIREJKO, L. A.: *Talyšsko-russkij slovar'*. Moskva 1976.

PLATTS 1930 = PLATTS, J. T.: *A dictionary of Urdū, classical Hindī, and English*. London[5] 1930.

POKORNY 1959 = POKORNY, J.: *Indogermanisches etymologisches Wörterbuch*. Vol. I-II. Bern 1959.

POHL 1981 = POHL, J.: 'Remarques sur la main, les doigts et la numération', in DE SIVERS 1981, 279–284.

POTT 1847 = POTT, A. F. : *Die quinare und vigesimale Zählmethode bei Völkern aller Welttheile. Nebst ausführlicheren Bemerkungen über die Zahlwörter indogermanischen Stammes und einem Anhang über Fingernamen*. Halle 1847.

PSTRUSIŃSKA 1974 = PSTRUSIŃSKA, J.: 'About the Origin of Comparison of Adjectives in Pashto', *Folia Orientalia* 15 (1974), 167–180.

PSTRUSIŃSKA 1985–1986 = PSTRUSIŃSKA, J.: 'The Influence of Linguistic Substratum on the Comparison of Adjectives in Pashto Language', *Folia Orientalia* 23 (1985–1986), 5–67.

PURHOSEYNI 1991 = PURHOSEYNI, A.: *Farhang-e loγāt va estelāhāt-e mardom-e Kermān*. Tehrān 1370/1991.

QAFISHEH 1997 = QAFISHEH, H.: *NTC's Gulf Arabic-English dictionary. A compact dictionary of the contemporary Arabic of the Mideast*. Lincolnwood (Chicago) 1997.

QALANDAR MOMAND – SEHRAYI 1994 = QALANDAR MOMAND – SEHRAYI, F.: *Pašto Luγat "Daryâb"*. 5 voll. Peshawar 1994.

RAHIMI – USPENSKAJA 1954 = RAHIMI, M. V. – USPENSKAJA, L. V., *Tadžiksko-russkij slovar'*. Moskva 1954.

RAHMĀNIĀN 2000 = RAHMĀNIĀN, D.: *Afsānehā-ye lori. Afsānehā-ye lori, baxtiāri va šuštari*. Tehrān 1379/2000.

RASTORGUEVA 1963 = RASTORGUEVA, V. S.: *Očerki po tadžikskoj dialektologii, 5. Tadžiksko-russkij dialektnyj slovar'*. Moskva 1963.

RAVĀQI 1995 = RAVĀQI, ᶜA.: *Qor'ān-e Qods. Kohantarin bargardān-e Qor'ān be fārsi?* 2 voll. Tehrān 1364/1995.

RAVERTY 1860 = RAVERTY, H. G.: *A dictionary of the Puk'hto, Pus'hto or Language of the Afghāns*. Hertford 1860.

RAXŠĀNI 1981 = RAXŠĀNI, B.: *Sistān. Jeld-e avval*. Tehrān 1360/1981.

RAZZAQ – BUKSH – FARRELL 2001 = RAZZAQ, A. – BUKSH, M. – FARRELL, T.: *Balochi Ganj. Balochi – English dictionary*. ms. (4th draft 2001).

REICHELT 1901 = REICHELT, H.: 'Der Frahang i Oīm (Zand-Pahlavi Glossary). Teil II', *Wiener Zeitschrift für die Kunde des Morgenlandes* 15 (1901), 117–186.

REDHOUSE 1968 = REDHOUSE, J.: *Redhouse yeni türkçe-inglizce sözlük / New Redhouse Turkish – English Dictionary*, İstanbul 1968.

REZĀI 1966 = REZĀI, J.: 'Farhang-e Mollā ᶜAli Ašraf-e Sabuhi be loγat-e ahl-e Birǰand', *Maǰalle-ye Dāneškāde-ye Adabiāt-e Dānešgāh-e Tehrān* 51/3 (1345/1966), 40–142.

REZĀI 1994 = REZĀI, J.: *Vāženāme-ye guyeš-e Birǰand*. Tehrān 1373/1994.

REZĀI 1998 = REZĀI, J.: *Barresi-e guyeš-e Birǰand*. Tehrān 1377/1998.

REZĀZĀDE MALEK 1973 = REZĀZĀDE MALEK, R.: *Guyeš-e āzari. Matn va tarǰome va vāženāme-ye resāle-ye Ruhi Anārǰāni.* (Entešārāt-e Anǰoman-e Irān-e Bāstān 6). Tehrān 1352/1973.

RIZGAR 1993 = RIZGAR, B.: *Kurdish-English, English-Kurdish* (*Kurmançî*) *dictionary / Ferheng Kurdî-Îngîlîzî, Îngîlîzî-Kurdî.* London 1993.

ROSSI 1979 = ROSSI, A. V.: *Iranian lexical elements in Brāhūī.* (Seminario di Studi Asiatici. Series Minor VIII). Naples 1979.

ROSSI 2002 = ROSSI, A. V.: 'Middle Iranian *gund* between Aramaic and Indo-Iranian', in *Studies in Honour of Shaul Shaked.* Jerusalem (= *Jerusalem Studies in Arabic and Islam*, 26 [2002]), 140–171.

ROSSI 2004–2006 = ROSSI, A. V.: 'Editorial Notes', *apud* B. FRAGNER, 'The disassembling of a European in Iran: An essay from Jalal Al-e Ahmad', *Balochistan Studies*, 11–12 (2004–2006), 49–69, [67–69].

ROZENFEL'D 1982 = ROZENFEL'D, A. Z: *Tadžiksko-russkij dialektnyj slovar'* (*jugo-vostočnyj Tadžikistan*). Leningrad 1982.

SĀDEQI 2000 = SĀDEQI, ᶜA. A.: *Negāh-i be guyešnāmehā-ye irāni* (*maǰmuᶜe-i az naqdhā va barresihā*). (Farhangestān-e zabān va adab-e fārsi. Markaz-e našr-e dānešgāhi 1009). Tehrān 1379/2000.

SĀDEQI 2001 = SĀDEQI, ᶜA. A.: *Fārsi-e qomi.* Tehrān 1380/2001.

SAFARI 1994 = SAFARI, H.: *Vāženāme-ye rāǰi. Guyeš-e šahrestān-e Deliǰān.* Tehrān 1373/1994.

SAFIZĀDE 2001 = SAFIZĀDE, S. (BURAKAI) : *Farhang-e Burakai-e kordi-fārsi.* 2 voll. Tehrān 1380/2001.

SALĀMI 2002 = SALĀMI, ᶜA.: *Farhang-e guyeš-e davāni.* (Farhangestān-e zabān va adab-e fārsi. Našr-e āsār 7). Tehrān 1381/2002.

SALĀMI 2004 = SALĀMI, ᶜA.: *Ganǰine-ye guyeš-šenāsi-e Fārs.* I. *Guyešhā-ye davāni, dahlei, ᶜabdui, kāzeruni, kalāni, kandei, kuzargi, mamassani, māsarmi.* (Farhangestān-e zabān va adab-e fārsi. Našr-e āsār 31). Tehrān 1383/2004.

SALĀMI 2005 = SALĀMI, ᶜA.: *Ganǰine-ye guyeš-šenāsi-e Fārs.* II. *Guyešhā-ye banāfi, pāpuni, dusirāni, riči, somγāni, kalāni (tāǰiki), gorganāi / gāvkošaki, mošqāni, nudāni.* (Farhangestān-e zabān va adab-e fārsi. Našr-e āsār 36). Tehrān 1384/2005.

SALĀMI 2006 = SALĀMI, ᶜA.: *Ganǰine-ye guyeš-šenāsi-e Fārs.* III. *Guyešhā-ye baliāni, birovakāni, hayāti (dowlatābādi), dādenǰāni, lor dārengāni, dorunaki / mehbudi, dežgāhi / guri, koroši, koruni.* (Farhangestān-e zabān va adab-e fārsi. Našr-e āsār 46). Tehrān 1385/2006.

SĀLEHI 1990 = SĀLEHI, S.: *Il-e bozorg-e baxtiāri* (*farhang-e vāžegān-e baxtiāri*). Tehrān 1369/1990.

SAMĀI 2003 = SAMĀI, M.: *Farhang-e loγāt-e zabān-e maxfi.* Tehrān 1382/2003.

SAMANDAR 1999 = SAMANDAR, B.: *Širāze az gol behtaru.* Tehrān 1378/1999.

SARLAK 2002 = SARLAK, R.: *Vāženāme-ye guyeš-e baxtiāri-e Čahār Lang.* (Farhangestān-e zabān va adab-e fārsi. Našr-e āsār 13). Tehrān 1381/2002.

SARYAZDI 2001 = SARYAZDI, M.: *Nāme-ye Sirǰān.* (Farhangestān-e zabān va adab-e fārsi. Našr-e āsār 5). Tehrān 1380/2001.

SAYAD HASHMI 2000 = SAYAD HASHMI: *Sayad Ganǰ.* Karāčī 2000.

SCERBO 1991 = SCERBO, E.: *Il nome della cosa. Nomi e nomignoli degli organi sessuali*. Milano 1991.

SCHIMMEL-ENDRES 1994 = SCHIMMEL, A. – ENDRES, F. C.: *The Mistery of Numbers*. Cambridge 1994.

SCHMITT 1989 = SCHMITT, R. (ed.): *Compendium Linguarum Iranicarum*. Wiesbaden 1989.

SCHWARTZ 1992 = SCHWARTZ, M.: 'On Proto-Indo-European **penk*^{w}- 'hand'', *Word* 43/3 (1992), 421–427.

SEPTFONDS 1994 = SEPTFONDS, D.: *Le Dzadrâni. Un parler pashto du Paktyâ* (*Afghanistan*). (Travaux de l'Institut d'Études Iraniennes de l'Université de la Sorbonne Nouvelle 15). Paris 1994.

SERRA 1971–1973 = SERRA, L.: 'Concordanze dialettali italiane con voci arabe e berbere e voci italiane in un dialetto berbero tripolitano', *Bollettino dell'Atlante Linguistico del Mediterraneo* 13–15 (1971–1973), 443–448.

SHAKED 1979 = SHAKED, Sh.: *The wisdom of the Sasanian sages (Dēnkard VI)*. (Persian Heritage Series 34). Boulder 1979.

SHAKED 1988 = SHAKED, Sh.: 'An early Geniza fragment in an unknown Iranian dialect', in *A Green Leaf. Papers in Honour of Professor Jes P. Asmussen*. (Acta Iranica 28. Deuxième série. Hommages et opera minora XII). Leiden 1988, 219–235.

SHAKED 2002 = SHAKED, Sh.: 'Towards a Middle Persian dictionary', in HUYSE, Ph. (ed.), *Iran. Questions et connaissances. Actes du IV*[e] *Congrès Européen des études iraniennes organisé par la Societas Iranologica Europaea Paris, 6–10 septembre 1999*. Vol. I. *La période ancienne*. (Studia Iranica – Cahier 25). Paris 2002, 120–134.

SHAKIBI-GUILANI – QOLIZADE VAZVANI 1990 = SHAKIBI-GUILANI, J. – QOLIZADE VAZVANI, M.: *A comparative probe in the Iranian dialects. 5. The Vajguni (The so-called Vazvani)*. Nashville 1990.

SHAKIBI-GUILANI – JAVAHERI 1993 = SHAKIBI-GUILANI, J. – JAVAHERI, M. H.: *A comparative probe in the Iranian dialects*. 14. *The Semnani dialects*. Nashville 1993.

SILVESTRI 2000 = SILVESTRI, D.: 'Dall'eloquenza della luce allo splendore della parola', *AIΩN. Annali del Dipartimento di Studi del Mondo Classico e del Mediterraneo Antico – Sezione linguistica* 22 (2000), 107–127.

SIMS-WILLIAMS 1983 = SIMS-WILLIAMS, N.: 'Chotano-Sogdica', *Bulletin of the School of Oriental and African Studies* 46 (1983), 40–51.

SIMS-WILLIAMS 1989 = SIMS-WILLIAMS, N.: 'A new fragment from the Parthian Hymn-Cycle *Huyadagmān*', in DE FOUCHÉCOUR, C.-H. – GIGNOUX, Ph. (eds.), *Études Irano-Aryennes offertes à Gilbert Lazard.* (Studia Iranica – Cahier 7). Paris 1989, pp. 321–331.

SIMS-WILLIAMS 2000 = SIMS-WILLIAMS, N.: *Bactrian documents from Northern Afghanistan* I. *Legal and economic documents*. Oxford 2000.

DE SIVERS 1979 = DE SIVERS, F. (éd.): *La main et les doigts dans l'expression linguistique*. (LACITO-documents – Eurasie 4). Paris 1979.

DE SIVERS 1981 = DE SIVERS, F. (éd.): *La main et les doigts dans l'expression linguistique II. Actes de la table ronde internationale du CNRS, Sèvres (France) 9–12 septembre 1980*. (LACITO-documents – Eurasie 6). Paris 1981.

SKJÆRVØ 1975 = SKJÆRVØ, P. O.: 'Notes on the dialects of Minab and Hormoz', *Norsk Tidsskrift for Sprogvidenskab* 29 (1975), 113–128.

SKJÆRVØ 1989 = SKJÆRVØ, P. O.: 'Pashto', in SCHMITT 1989, 384–410.

SKÖLD 1936 = SKÖLD, H.: *Materialien zu den iranischen Pamirsprachen*. Wörterverzeichnisse von H. SMITH. (Skrifter utgivna av kungl. humanistika vetenskapssamfundet i Lund XXI). Lund 1936.

SOHRĀBI ANĀRAKI 1994 = SOHRĀBI ANĀRAKI, A.: *Vāženāme-ye anāraki*. Mašhad 1373/1994.

SOKOLOVA 1959 = SOKOLOVA, V. S.: *Rušanskie i xufskie teksty i slovar'*. Moskva – Leningrad 1959.

SORUŠIĀN 1956 = SORUŠIĀN, M. S.: *Farhang-e behdinān*, ed. by M. SOTUDE. Tehrān 1956 (recent repr. 1370/1991).

SOTUDE 1957 = SOTUDE, M.: *Farhang-e kermāni*.(Entešārāt-e Farhang-e Irānzamin 4). Tehrān 1335/1957.

SOTUDE 1958 = SOTUDE, M.: 'Xoini. Yeki az lahǰehā-ye āzari', *Farhang-e Irānzamin* 6 (1337/1958), 324–327.

SOTUDE 1962 = SOTUDE, M.: 'Lahǰe-ye ᶜAli Ābād-e Farim', *Farhang-e Irānzamin* 10 (1341/1962), 437–470.

SOTUDE 1963 = SOTUDE, M.: *Farhang-e semnāni, sorxei, lāsgardi, sangsari, šahmerzādi*. (Entešārāt-e Dānešgāh-e Tehrān 883). Tehrān 1342/1963.

SOTUDE 1986 = SOTUDE, M.: *Farhang-e nāini*. (Mo'assese-ye motāleᶜāt va tahqiqāt-e farhangi 559). Tehrān 1375/1986.

SOTUDE 1989 = SOTUDE, M.: 'Vāžehāi az zabān-e mardom-e Nehāvand', *Farhang-e Irānzamin* 28 (1368/1989), pp. 70–78.

STEBLIN-KAMENSKIJ 1999 = STEBLIN-KAMENSKIJ, I. M.: *Ėtimologičeskij slovar' vaxanskogo jazyka*. Sankt-Peterburg 1999.

STEINGASS 1963 = STEINGASS, F.: *A comprehensive Persian-English dictionary*. London[5] 1963 [first ed. 1892].

STILO 2004 = STILO, D. L.: *Vafsi folk tales. Twenty four folk tales in the Gurchani dialect of Vafsi as narrated by Ghazanfar Mahmudi and Mashdi Mahdi and collected by L. P. ELWELL-SUTTON*. Transcribed, translated and annotated by D. L. STILO. Supplied with folkloristik notes and edited by U. MARZOLPH. (Beiträge zur Iranistik 25). Wiesbaden 2004.

STILO 2007 = STILO, D.: 'Isfahan. xxi. Provincial Dialects', in *Encyclopædia Iranica* XIV. (Ed. by E. YARSHATER). New York 2007, 93–112.

STRAZHAS 1979 = STRAZHAS, N.: 'Contrastive Studies of the "hand" and the "finger" in English, Russian and Lithuanian', in DE SIVERS 1979, 67–71.

SUNDERMANN 1994 = SUNDERMANN, W.: 'Manohmed rōšn "der Licht-Nous". Ursprung und Wandel eines manichäischen Begriffs', in RÖHRBORN, K. – VEENKER, W. (eds.), *Memoriae Munusculum. Gedenkband für Annemarie von Gabain*. Wiesbaden 1994, 123–129 [reprinted in RECK, Ch. – WEBER, D. – LEURINI, C. –PANAINO, A. (eds.), *Manichaica Iranica. Ausgewählte Schriften von Werner Sundermann*. 2 voll. (Serie Orientale Roma LXXXIX, 1–2). Roma 2001, 587–594].

SUNDERMANN 2002 = SUNDERMANN, W.: ' 'The Book of the Head' and 'The Book of the Limb'. A Sogdian Word List', in HUYSE, Ph. (ed.), *Iran. Questions et connaissances. Actes du IVᵉ Congrès Européen des études iraniennes organisé par la Societas Iranologica Europaea Paris, 6–10 septembre 1999*. Vol. I. *La période ancienne*. (Studia Iranica – Cahier 25). Paris 2002, 135–161.

SUNDERMANN 2003 = SUNDERMANN, W.: 'Notulae Etymologicae', in VAN TONGERLOO, A. (ed.), *Iranica Selecta. Studies in honour of Professor Wojciech Skalmowski on the occasion of his seventieth birthday*. (Silk Road Studies VIII). Turnhout 2003, 219–224.

SZEMERÉNYI 1971 = SZEMERÉNYI, O.: Review of CHANTRAINE, P., *Dictionnaire étymologique de la langue grecque*. I-II. Paris 1970, *Gnomon* 43 (1971), 641–675.

SZEMERÉNYI 1977 = SZEMERÉNYI, O.: 'Studies in the kinship terminology of the Indo-European languages', in *Varia 1977*. (Acta Iranica 16. Troisième série. Textes et mémoires VII). Leiden, 1–240.

ŠĀLČI 1991 = ŠĀLČI, A.: *Farhang-e guyeš-e Xorāsān-e bozorg*. Tehrān 1370/1991.

ŠĀMLU 2000 ŠĀMLU, A. *Ketāb-e kuče* III. *Harf-e Alef, daftar-e dovvom*. Tehrān 1379/2000.

ŠARI[c]ATZÂDE 1992 = ŠARI[c]ATZÂDE, Seyyed [c]A. A.: *Farhang-e mardom-e Šāhrud*. Tehrān 1371/1992.

ŠĀYEGĀN 2006 = ŠĀYEGĀN, M.: *Vāženāme-ye guyeš-e xuri*. Tehrān 1385/2006.

ŠOKRI 1995 = ŠOKRI, G.: *Guyeš-e sāri* (*māzandarāni*). (Pežuhešgāh-e [c]olum-e ensāni va motālehāt-e farhangi 553). Tehrān 1374/1995.

ŠOKRI 2006 = ŠOKRI, G.: *Guyeš-e rāmsari*. (Pežuhešgāh-e [c]olum-e ensāni va motālehāt-e farhangi). Tehrān 1385/2006.

TA[c]DĀDI SANGESARI 2002 = TA[c]DĀDI SANGESARI, F.: *Adabiāt-e [c]āmiāne-ye Sangesar*. Tehrān 1381/2002.

TAKAZOV 2003 = TAKAZOV, F. M.: *Digoron-urussag Dzurduat / Digorsko-russkij slovar'*. Vladikavkaz 2003.

TĀRIQ MĀLISTĀNI 1993= TĀRIQ MĀLISTĀNI, A. H.: *Farhang-e ebtedāi-ye melli-ye hazāra. Be enzemām-e tarǰome be fārsi-englisi / Hazaragi-Dari/Farsi-English. A preliminary glossary*. Koetta 1993.

TAVADIA 1930 = TAVADIA, J. C.: *Šāyast nē Šāyast. A Pahlavi text on religious customs*. Edited, transliterated and translated with introduction and notes by J. C TAVADIA. (Alt- und Neu-Indische Studien 3). Hamburg 1930.

TAVERNIER 2007 = TAVERNIER, J.: *Iranica in the Achaemenid period (ca. 550–330 B.C.). Lexicon of Old Iranian proper names and loanwords, attested in Non-Iranian Texts*. (Orientalia Lovaniensia Analecta 158). Leuven 2007.

TĀVUSI 1986 = TĀVUSI, M.: *Vāženāme-ye Šāyest našāyest*. (Entešārāt-e Dānešgāh-e Širāz 130). Širāz 1365/1986.

TEDESCO 1921 = TEDESCO, P.: 'Dialektologie der westiranischen Turfantexte', *Le Monde Oriental* 15 (1921) 184–258.

THOMAS 1930 = THOMAS, B.: 'The Kumzari dialect of Shihuh Tribe, Arabia, and a vocabulary', *Journal of the Royal Asiatic Society* (1930), 785–854.

THOMAS 1981 = THOMAS, J. M. C.: 'La main et les doigts dans l'expression linguistique de quelques langues d'Afrique Centrale', in DE SIVERS 1981, 335–351.

TODD 1985 = TODD, T.: *A Grammar of Dimilī (also known as Zaza)*. PhD diss., The University of Michigan. Ann Arbor (UMI) 1985.

TOMASCHEK 1880 = TOMASCHEK, W.: 'Centralasiatische Studien II. Die Pamir-Dialekte', *Sitzunberichte der Wiener Akad. d. Wissensch., phil.-hist. Kl.* 96 (1880), 735–900.

TREMBLAY 2000 = TREMBLAY, X.: Review of R. E. EMMERICK – P. O. SKJÆRVØ, *Studies in the Vocabulary of Khotanese* III. (Sitzungsberichte der Österreichischen Akademie der Wissenschaften. Philosophisch-historische Klasse, 651 / Veröffentlichungen der Iranischen Kommission 27). Wien 1997, *Indo-Iranian Journal* 43 (2000), 191–196.

TREMBLAY 2005 = TREMBLAY, X.: Review of MORGENSTIERNE 2003, *Bulletin de la Société de Linguistique* 100 (2005), 173–184.

TURNER 1966 TURNER, R. L.: *A Comparative Dictionary of the Indo-Aryan Languages*. London 1966.

UNVALA 1958 = UNVALA, J. M.: 'Contributions to modern Persian dialectology. The Lurī and Dizfūlī dialects. II', *Indo-Iranica* 11/4 (1958), 1–16.

UTAS – NYBERG 1988 = UTAS, B. (ed.) : *Frahang i Pahlavīk*, edited with transliteration, transcription and commentary from the posthumous papers of Henrik Samuel NYBERG, with the collaboration of Christopher TOLL. Wiesbaden 1988.

VAHMAN 1886 = VAHMAN, F.: *Ardā Wīrāz Nāmag. The Iranian "Divina Comedia"*. (Scandinavian Institute of Asian Studies Monograph Series 53). London 1986.

VAHMAN – ASATRIAN 1987 = VAHMAN, F. – ASATRIAN, G.S.: *West Iranian Dialect Materials from the collection of D. L. Lorimer*. Vol. I. *Materials on the Ethnography of the Baxtiārīs. Introduction, texts, translation, glossary & notes*. (Series of Iranian Studies I). Copenhagen 1987.

VAHMAN – ASATRIAN 1999 = VAHMAN, F. – ASATRIAN, G.: 'Gleanings from Zāzā Vocabulary', in *Iranica Varia. Papers in Honor of Prof. E. Yarshater*. (Acta Iranica 30. Troisième série. Textes et mémoires XVI). Leiden 1999, 267–275.

VAHMAN – ASATRIAN 2002 = VAHMAN, F. – ASATRIAN, G.: *Notes on the Language and Ethnography of the Zoroastrians of Yazd*. (Historisk-filosofiske Meddelelser 85). Copenhagen 2002.

VEENKER 1981 = VEENKER, W.: 'Einige Besonderheiten in der Benennung der Finger in verschiedenen Sprachen des eurasischen Areals', in DE SIVERS 1981, 361–376.

WAAG 1941 = WAAG, A.: *Nirangistan. Der Awestatraktat über die rituellen Vorschriften*. (Iranische Forschungen 2). Leipzig 1941.

WAHBY – EDMONDS 1966 = WAHBY, T. – EDMONDS, C. J.: *A Kurdish-English dictionary*. Oxford 1966.

WEHR 1979 = WEHR, H.: *A dictionary of modern written Arabic* (*Arabic-English*). Ed. by J. MILTON COWAN. Fourth edition considerably enlarged and emended by the author. Wiesbaden 1979.

WILLIAMS 1990 = WILLIAMS, A. V.: *The Pahlavi Rivāyat accompanying the Dādestān ī Dēnīg*. Part I: *Transliteration, transcription and glossary*. Part II:

Translation, commentary and Pahlavi text. (Historisk-filosofiske Meddelelser 60: 1–2). Copenhagen 1990.

WINDFUHR 1995 = WINDFUHR, G. L.: 'Dialectology', in *Encyclopædia Iranica* VII. (Ed. by E. YARSHATER). Costa Mesa 1995, 362–370.

XADIŠ 2000 = XADIŠ, H.: *Farhang-e mardom-e Širāz.* Širāz 1379/2000.

XASRAVI 1989 = XASRAVI, ᶜA. (QĀED-E BAXTIĀRI): *Farhang-e baxtiāri.* Tehrān 1368/1989.

XAZDUZ 2002 = XADZUZ, M.: *Kāku-ye širāzi.* Širāz 1381/2002.

XROMOV 1972 = XROMOV, A. L.: *Jagnobskij jazyk.* Moskva 1972.

YARSHATER 1969 = YARSHATER, E.: *A grammar of Southern Tati dialects.* (Median Dialect Studies I). The Hague – Paris 1969.

YARSHATER 2001 = YARSHATER, E.: '"A Peasant Marriage", a Poem in Chāli by Moḥammad-Bāqer ᶜĀmeli', *Studia Iranica* 30 (2001), 245–289.

YÜCE – BENZING 1985 = YÜCE, N. – BENZING, J.: 'Khwarezmische Wörter und Sätze einer choresmtürkischen Handschrift der Muqaddimat al-Adab', *Zeitschrift der Deutschen Morgenländischen Gesellschaft* 135 (1985), 92–103.

ZAND MOQADDAM 1991 = ZAND MOQADDAM, M.: *Hekāyate Baloč* I. Tehrān 1370/1991.

ZARUBIN 1960 = ZARUBIN, I. I.: *Šugnanskie teksty i slovar'.* Moskva – Leningrad 1960.

ZIĀN 1960 = ZIĀN, J.: 'Lahǰe-ye sivandi', *Maǰalle-ye Dāneškade-ye Adabiāt-e Širāz*, 3/5 (1339/1960), 61–91.

ZOMORRODIĀN 1989 = ZOMORRODIĀN, R.: *Barresi-e guyeš-e Qāin.* Ostān-e Qods-e Rezavi 1368/1989.

ZOKĀ 1954 = ZOKĀ, I.: *Guyeš-e Keringān* (*tāti*). Tehrān 1332/1954.

ZVELEBIL 1985 = ZVELEBIL, K. V.: 'The Body in Nilgiri Tribal Languages. A Contribution to Areal Linguistic Studies', *Journal of the American Oriental Society* 105/4 (1985), 653–674.

ŽUKOVSKIJ 1888 = ŽUKOVSKIJ, V. A.: *Materialy dlja izučenija persidskix" naréčij.* I. *Dialekty polosy goroda Kašana: Vonišun", Koxrud", Kešė, Zėfrė.* Sanktpeterburg" 1888.

ŽUKOVSKIJ 1922 = ŽUKOVSKIJ, V. A.: *Materialy dlja izučenija persidskix" naréčij.* II. *Dialekty goroda Semnana: Sėngisėr", Šemerzod". Dialekty polosy goroda Isfagana: Sėdė, Gjaz", Kjafron". Dialekty polosy goroda Širaza: Sivend", Abdui. Guranskij dialekt" derevni Talaxedĕšk". Naréčie evreev" goroda Kašana. Naréčie derevni Tadžriš".* I *Teksty*, II *Slovar'*. Petrograd" 1922.

CHAPTER ONE: INTRODUCTION

1. Fingers have a prominent position in everyday experience and in the perception people have of human body. They are natural instruments for ordinary actions. With fingers people point, touch, press, scratch, grasp, tighten, beat, tap, count, and so on. When people look at their own body, fingers and hands, being generally uncovered, are the first parts to be perceived; when people look at other people, they are generally the second, immediately after the face.

Fingers, like people, are individually animated, i.e., all fingers can move separately and autonomously and their movement is extremely eye-catching. People often accompany their talking with movements of their hands and fingers, regardless of the topic and in many cases unconsciously, though with different modalities according to the cultural system they belong to and their individual background.

A human hand has five fingers, and computation by means of fingers has proved to be a universal computational strategy.[3] How counting as a cognitive ability has originated, which are the relationships between enumeration, cognition and cultures, how numerals have been conceptualized and verbalized, etc. are very complex questions, out of my present interests.[4] I will spend here only a few words, which may prove useful to further steps in our investigation, without going into details.

It is certain that the human body in general, and hands and fingers in particular, have had a relevant function in the establishment of numerical systems. However, different ways of conceptualization may have parallelly existed and competed each other, generating linguistic stratifications in one and the same linguistic/cultural environment (GNERRE 1995).

The different computational strategies with basis '4', '5', '10' and '20', some of which may have coexisted at certain times, can all be explained resorting to the natural usage of hands (and in some cases feet) by human people. The bases '5', '10' and '20' are self-explanatory, being equivalent to the

---

3 Cf. POHL 1981: 284, LANDI 2000, EDELMAN 1999: 229.

4 The bibliography on the matter is so rich, that quoting it *in extenso* is not possible. A collection of papers on the subject, with the relevant bibliography, presented on the occasion of the International Conference on "Numeri e istanze di numerazione tra preistoria e protostoria linguistica del mondo antico" (Naples, 1–2 December 1995) is in *AIΩN* 17 (1995).

totality of the fingers of one hand, of two hands and of the digits in a human body, respectively. The basis '4' could be considered as less transparent at first. To a quartal system resorted HENNING (1948) interpreting the Ir. word for '8' as a dual form of Av. *ašti-* '(a measure of length) four finger's breadth, palm'. Similarly, the Hittite word for '4', *mieu-*, *miu-* (< IE **mei-* 'to lessen; to be small'), has been interpreted as derived from the designation of the "little hand" (the hand with the exclusion of the thumb).[5] The latter derivation was challenged by GNERRE (1995: 149), who prefers an explanation based on the lunar mansions. In fact, he considers the "little hand" hypothesis as possible, but unprovable («al momento non conosco dati etnografici che appoggino una tale ipotesi, ed una percezione (ed uso) della mano di questo tipo»).

Both Iranian and IA, however, bear witness to the fact that the four fingers from the index to the little finger may be perceived as an independent concept. Beside Av. *ašti-* quoted above, we have Yγn. *paxa*, explained as 'the four finger of the hand (with the exclusion of the thumb)'[6] in XROMOV 1972, Skt. *catur aṅgulá* 'the four fingers of the hand (without the thumb); 4 finger broad, 4 inches' and the several equivalent expressions in Ir. languages, pointing to a unitary concept. These are Sgl. *čāraŋgešt*, Išk. *čor-angĭšt* 'span, from thumb to fore-finger', Šγn. *čōr-angux̌t/angix̌t*, Baǰ. *čōr-ingax̌t* 'a measure of length, from the forefinger to the little finger' ('the distance between the thumb and the ring finger' ZARUBIN 1960), Yzγ. *čorangəx̌t* 'the measure of length corresponding to four stretched fingers', Rod. *čahār angošt* 'the distance between the four fingers, the thumb excluded [*fāsele-ye beyn-e čahār angošt manhā-ye angošt-e šast*]' (MOᶜTAMEDI 2001: 171), AfγPrs. (Her.) *čâr angošt* 'a measure of length a little smaller than a span', etc. In Colloquial Prs., *čahār angošt* is used to mean 'very small', 'having a very small dimension' (NAJAFI 1999).

Even by the following Prs. passage: *pesar čahār angošt-aš rā yek-i kard va* [...] *be surat-e doxtar zad* ("the boy joined his four fingers and [...] hit the girl's face"), extrapolated from a tale published in BEHRANGI – DEHQĀNI 1969: 142, we may infer that *čahār angošt* is (or may be) perceived as a unitary concept in Persian.[7]

---

5 For bibliographical references see GNERRE 1995: 148–149 and fn. 30.

6 On Yγn. *pax, paxa* see below, pp. 70 ff.

7 Note the pronominal suffix *-aš* and the definite/specific object marker *rā*, which points to an already introduced or otherwise, as in this case, definite object.

There are several etymologies for the IE words for 'five'.[8] The one proposed by HOROWITZ (1992) and supported by SCHWARTZ (1992), points to IE *$penk^w$-* as the original IE word for 'hand'; once this base had been incorporated into the numerical system for 'five', it was replaced in later phases of the IE languages by other words for 'hand'. This fact could provide, according to HOROWITZ, a satisfactory explanation for the lacking of a common IE word for this very salient body part.[9] The conceptual association underlying the alleged phenomenon would not differ from the more recent one which produced Tafr. *dost* 'number ten' (ADIB TUSI 1963–1964) by means of a semantic extension from 'hand(s)', and Yγn. *paxxa* 'ten, tenner' (MIRZOZODA 2008, s.v. *paxxa*[3]) by means of a semantic extension from 'finger(s)'.

To conclude this digression into the numerical domain, one may note that the number five has been regarded in several different cultures as THE PERFECT NUMBER, the number of completeness (see e.g. CREVATIN 1978: 7-11) and that the pentad has been perceived as a CANONICAL SET (SCHWARTZ 1992: 424).[10] This finds an explanation in the fact that the fingers, which as a whole constitute a hand and represent a totality, are five in all. Examples from Persian classical poetry testify the symbolic value of FIVE. A clear instance is the case of 'five days' equated to TOTALITY OF LIFE (MOKRI 2005: 269–270).

2. The potential of hands and fingers is magnified by the symbolic power which human people universally attribute to them. With a simple movement of the hand or of a single finger one may give order, greet, bless, accuse, curse, insult; one may swear, nullify his own oath, pledge, attest one's own identity, testify one's own faith, contract alliances, reinforce social hierarchies, etc.; using a well established gestural code one may send every kind of messages. This makes the hand and the fingers highly powerful and dangerous performative organs. Since ancient times, both positive and negative

---

8 See a collection of them in BLAŽEK 2000.

9 For a different explanation, see § 2 below.

10 Cf. Prs. *dast* 'hand' used in the sense of 'set' (*yekdast lebās* 'suit'; *yek dast bošqāb* 'a set of plates', etc.). I take the opportunity to signal here what could be an apparently odd usage of *dast* ('hand') in the AfγPrs. dialect of Herat, which contrasts with what one would normally expect. Besides being used as a numerative for clothes, Her. *dast* is also recorded with the meaning of 'six of anything'; we can probably envisage here a reflex of what is the traditionally accepted concept of PERFECT NUMBER, which varies according to different objects.

powers have been attributed to them in culturally and geographically different areas.[11] As it happens to eyes, fingers are conceived as endowed with the magic power of casting a spell on someone in order to drive out evil. Well known in the Islamic world is the apotropaic function of the open hand showed to the enemy, symbolized by the famous hand-shaped amulet called *xams* (< 'five'), also known as "the hand of Fatima", a real "symbole d'accompagnement" in the Maghrebine tradition according to CHEBEL 1999: 86, widespread in all the Middle East and North Africa.[12] The very gesture of stretching one's hand against someone's face, or the simple word *xams* 'five' is understood as a very dangerous curse (SCHIMMEL – ENDRES 1994: 115–116). In Iranian, Xuns. *penǰa* and Bal. *panč* (from 'five', see below pp. 76 ff.), recorded as 'curse made with the open hand, showing the palm towards someone's face', also attest the aggressive power of this gesture. The potential dangerousness of hands and fingers could have generated linguistic taboos; BONFANTE (1939) explains in these terms the lack of IE common words for 'hand',[13] and even more for 'finger'.

3. For their shape and their functioning as sexual surrogates, the fingers are frequently equated to the male sexual organ. SCERBO (1991: 47, 48) describes as follows the metaphorical mapping FINGER = MALE ORGAN in European languages: «Nei paesi di lingua francese, oltre a *doigt* [..] "dito", considerato simbolo del pene, sono diffuse le seguenti metafore: *le doigt medium,* ovvero *le doigt de milieu,* "il dito di mezzo", cioè quello posto fra le gambe dell'uomo; *le doigt que n'a pas d'ongle* [...] In alcune canzoni anonime troviamo la metafora *brigadier de l'amour* nel significato di "dito medio" per l'assistenza che tale dito offre nei giochi erotici [...] in Francia il dito medio della mano destra è chiamato anche *doigt de la cour* "dito cortigiano". [...] Fra le popolazioni di lingua inglese si registrano con lo stesso significato le seguenti denominazioni: *little finger* [...], *forefinger* [...], *thumb of love* [...], *middle finger* [...]». Similarly, *angošt-e šekam*, lit. 'the finger of

---

11 References to an "evil finger" (*ubânu limuttim*) and a "good finger" (*ubânu damiqtim*) in the Akkadian world are in EBELING 1957. On the magic power attributed to hands and fingers see also BONFANTE 1939: 202–203 and BRACCHI 2009: 281–286.

12 On the symbolism of the hand in the Islamic (mainly Arabic) world see CHEBEL 1995, s.vv. *Khoms, Main, Doigts, Phalange* (with relevant bibliography); CHEBEL 1999: 85–90. Prs. *xamse-ye mobāreke* 'the fingers (the five prospering (blessed) ones)' (STEINGASS 1963) also points to the special protective function of the hand. On the symbolism and the magic potential of the number five see SCHIMMEL – ENDRES 1994: 105–121.

13 For a different explanation see § 1 above.

the belly', *angošt-e bist-o-yekom*, lit. 'the twenty-first finger' (ŠĀMLU 2000: 1018) are (jesting) alternative expressions for the male organ in Persian.

The finger as a metaphor of the male genital organ is a recognized universal which finds an explanation not only in the finger's shape and its possible practical usages: in many cultures, fingers and hands are regarded as conceptually linked with the human procreative power, as underlined by ONIANS (1998: 231–232 fn. 9, 276 fn. 2, 356–359) as far as the Classical and Hebrew worlds are concerned. In this light, one should probably explain the Phl. expression *dast-hušk* 'dried hand(s)', occurring for example in *Dk.* V, 2.3, where we are told in which way the *dev*s, who have tried to make Zardušt die, were punished (*kē margīh kē agārīh ud tā-z kē dast hušk* "Certains (d'entre eux) furent atteints par la mort et d'autres (rendus) impuissants, à telle enseigne que leurs mains se desséchèrent", AMOUZGAR – TAFAZZOLI 2000: 26–27).[14]

In order to establish a new etymology for Av. *zasta-* 'hand' (and its several cognates), GERSHEVITCH (1996) reconstructs a root **ĝhes-* 'to extend', to which he also refers Av. *āžu-*, Sgd. *''ẓw* 'penis (probably only in expanded size)'. In this way, he suggests an etymological link between *zasta-* 'hand' (*zas-ta-*) 'the extendible' and Gath. *āžu-* 'penis' (*ā-ž-*(*u*)-) 'the expansive'. I will straddle here the issue of the likelihood of GERSHEVITCH' proposal; I am sure, however, he would have rejoiced to know that witness to the equivalence HAND = MALE ORGAN is born at least by Nāi. *das* 'hand; male organ' (also Krmnš. *das-e xar* 'male genital organ (vulg.)').

Being associated to the male organ, fingers are also capable of evoking obscene concepts. Therefore, obscene senses are frequently associated to labels for fingers; cf. Engl. *finger*, as in the idiom *giving someone the finger*, referring to the obscene gesture (also known as *bird*) made by extending the middle finger while bending the other fingers into the palm, which is very common in several areas in the world, including the ones we are concerned with here. The practice to do obscene gestures with fingers to abuse someone by sending him messages with clear sexual contents is a universal.[15] Which

---

14 See also *Dk.* VII 3.6 (MOLÉ 1993: 170), *WZ* 10.3 (GIGNOUX – TAFAZZOLI 1993: 66–67). On the other hand, one could interpret as originally meaning 'endowed with procreative powers' the Prs. idiom *tar-dast* 'dexterous' (lit. 'wet-handed'), already attestd in Phl. (cf. SHAKED 2002: 132–133).

15 The relevant Ir. linguistic expressions which may be put forward in this connection are numberless. I will limit myself to quote here, as a sample of the different possibilities, Zar. *nâxû nœšû* 'dishonoured, infamous, disgraced', which may be said of a person to which a finger (*nâxû*) has been shown; Zarq. *angol dādan* 'to insult with a gesture made

finger(s) to use for this purpose, and in which way, depends on the different cultural traditions; the middle finger and the thumb generally compete for such a role. The ancient Romans, for example, used the middle finger;[16] in Iran, showing the thumb while keeping the other fingers bent is not exactly a mark of friendship. A held up thumb is perceived as a deliberately aggressive gesture in the IA[17] and Drav. areas[18], as well. For the Baloch, the sticking up of the middle finger or its bending downwards while keeping the other fingers straight forwards transmit obscene messages; in some areas of Balochistan, however, it is the thumb that carries out this task. The erotic potential of the fingers increases the perception of their salutariness and/or dangerousness.

4. Most of the matters just hinted at so far about the position of the hand and the fingers in human imagery, their ordinary functions, their symbolic value, their role in substaining devotional and ideological systems, their capacity to communicate, etc. lie at the intersection of a large number of scientific fields (semiotics, cognitive semantics, cognitive ethnography, anthropology, psychology, iconography, etc.). Two International Round Tables, organized respectively in Ivry and Sèvres in 1978 and 1980 by the French CNRS, had as their subject "La main et les doigts dans l'expression linguistique". The collections of the papers presented at the two meetings (DE SIVERS 1979, 1981) clearly show the diversity of domains, methodologies and interests which «l'étude des rapports entre la pensée et la main» (DE SIVERS 1979: 1) may involve.

---

showing one of one's own fingers (and in particular the forefinger) to someone else, with the nail in the direction of the insulted person (also to deceive, trick)'; Bal. *gaḍḍī kanag* 'to stick one's finger up (either physically poking someone from behind with the middle finger, or sticking this finger in the air as a sign of abuse. Very impolite)' and by semantic extension, 'to fiddle with, to mess with' (RAZZAQ – BUKSH – FARRELL 2001); Damāv. *hāppās* 'to insult someone, showing the thumb, sometimes after having insalivated it'. On THUMB = MALE ORGAN cf. also Prs. *šast* ('thumb') and its derivative *šastak* 'dildo', recorded by in traditional dictionaries (see DEHX). On the sexual value attached to the thumb in the ancient Roman world, see ONIANS 1998: 561 and fn. 4.

16 POTT (1847: 288–291) provides a rich documentation on a few Lat. names of the middle finger (such as *digitus infamis* (or *famosus*), *digitus impudicus* etc.) that find their motivation on the association with the male sexual organ.

17 Cf. CDIAL 5506, 5515.

18 Cf. DED^2 4425.

The aim of the present work is to analyse in a motivational perspective[19] all the words for 'finger' and the names of individual fingers in the Iranian languages, reconstructing in this way an iconomastic typology for the 'finger' lexical domain in Iranian. In the framework of modern onomasiology, which operates in the light of cognitive linguistics, I concentrated on the 'pathways' through which the concept FINGER in general and those for individual fingers have been verbalized, going back (when possible) to the respective source concepts. Many regularities in the recurrent schemas have been proved to exist, some of which are universal, being present not only in Iranian or areally connected languages, but also in languages not related at all. At the same time, through occasional sorties in conceptual domains other than FINGER, which have given the opportunity of several cross-linguistic semasiological digressions, I intended contributing a little to the general knowledge of Iranian lexicon, which, despite the outstanding work of great scholars in the past two centuries, still remains a neglected branch of Iranology.

Bibliographical references on items having as subject the names of the individual fingers are MOINFAR 1981: 230 (Persian; only "standard" names), FILIPPONE 2000–2003 (Balochi), MOKRI 2005: 262–264 (Persian). A very important collection of finger names in many languages of the world is in POTT 1847: 225–304 ('Anhang über Fingernamen'), which still remains of great interest and contains a very rich documentation for Iranian.

5. The upper and lower human body limbs have five endings each, in a sense similar in shape, which are free and mobile. The whole of the five digits can be conceptualized as a unit, and can be verbalized with a specific word. This is what happens, for example, in languages like Persian, where the term *panǰe*, a derivative from *panǰ* 'five', denotes 'the five digits as a whole' and consequently the 'hand' (or the 'foot');[20] it lays emphasis upon the salience of the five digits at the ending of the body limbs.

---

19 Motivation is intended here as a fundamental component of the linguistic sign, autonomous with respect both to meaning and etymology, according to the lines outlined by ALINEI (1996). ALINEI has also been the first to introduce terms like *iconimo*, *iconimologia*, *iconomastica*, etc., which are used in the present book in their English form (iconym, iconomastic etc.). In 2005, *Quaderni di semantica*, Bologna, the journal edited by ALINEI, changed its original subtitle (*Rivista internazionale di semantica teorica e applicata / An International Journal of Theoretical and Applied Semantics*) into *Rivista internazionale di semantica e iconomastica / An International Journal of Semantics and Iconomastics*.

20 For more details see below pp. 76 ff.

There are languages that differentiate lexically the endings of the hand from those of the foot. English, for example, has *finger* and *toe*, German has *Finger* and *Zehe*, French has *doigt* and *orteil*. There are languages in which FINGER and TOE have been verbalized as a unique concept (DIGIT). Among these, one may count the Ir. languages. If required by the context, the relevant term may be specified as 'pertaining to the hand', or 'to the foot'; in Persian, for example, *angošt-e dast* 'finger' (lit. 'the digit of the hand') contrasts with *angošt-e pā* 'toe' (lit. 'the digit of the foot'). In Iranian, exceptions to this general assumption are few, if any: all of them could be easily explained as the result either of partially wrong analyses by modern Western scholars, influenced by a categorization typical of their own languages (as is the case of Av. *angušta-* 'toe', see below, p. 56), or of a recategorization of original lexical hierarchies by native speakers living abroad (as could be the case with the discordant distinctions proposed in some Kurdish bilingual dictionaries published in Europe, see below, p. 85).

Given the salience of the fingers in everyday human experience, as compared to that of the toes, in what follows I will always refer to 'finger' (if not otherwise specified). Note that, though words for 'finger' may be used with reference to the toe, the automatic application of individual finger names to the corresponding toes is not (or not always) possible, as demonstrated for Balochi in FILIPPONE 2000–2003: 72–73. Since an adequate lexicographic documentation on the matter lacks, I will concentrate on the finger names, leaving off the toe names.

Finger names may consist of single words or may be lexicalized phrases, generally containing two lexical units, the second being 'finger', whose presence may be or not be indispensable. In some cases the motivations underlying them are no longer obvious; in other cases they are still transparent and the speaker is able to recognize the associative connections that have produced those specific names. As a consequence of the general trend towards standardization in the major Ir. languages, a wealth of terms for individual fingers with an interesting cultural motivation has been replaced by one more or less official name.[21]

---

[21] This is a common phenomenon, involving all linguistic areas. It is in this light that one should reconsider the data offered by cross-language researches, like those presented in BROWN – WITKOWSKI 1981, concerning the presence of figurative names for certain body parts. In particular, with regard to figurative expressions for fingers and toes, it is stated that they are extremely rare in European languages, which «do not use figurative language in naming these body parts» (p. 601). This comment has been biased by the sources used for each language involved in their analysis (118 languages in all), characterized by dif-

6. Finger names have a marked status and are low in salience; consequently they have a very low frequency in both everyday speech and written texts. Nevertheless almost everybody learns the traditional finger names very early in life, often in association with nursery-rhymes, which folk repertoires generally abound with. There are finger rhymes telling no story but consisting of the finger names uttered one after the other; some instances in Balochi are provided below, p. 140. There are finger rhymes depicting the fingers as having active roles in actions (mainly escapades) and dialogues. In these cases, the fingers may or may not be referred to by means of their names; the mentioning of the fingers is usually accompanied by touching them in turn.[22] Most people (children and adults) in Tehran and surroundings seem to know the rhyme entitled *lili howzak*; several variants of this popular Prs. rhyme exist elsewhere (a Her. version is quoted in ĀSEF FEKRAT 1997, s.v.). The initial event on which the matter turns is the falling of something (a goat) in a *howzak*, a small water basin (the hollow of the palm of one's own hand perfectly meets the case). In a different rhyme, the fingers are portrayed as planning a theft. The following are respectively (a) a Prs. version I recorded in Tehran and (b) a similar Semn. version, published in MORGENSTIERNE 1960: 77–78:

(a)

little f.	*in mige berim bedozdim*	"this one says: let's go thieving"
ring f.	*in mige či bedozdim*	"this one says: what should we thieve?"
middle f.	*in mige tašt-e talā bedozdim*	"this one says: let's thieve a gold cup"
foref.	*in mige ǰavāb-e xodā ro či bedim?*	"this one say: what answer shall we give to God?"
thumb	*in mige man-e man-e kalle gonde*	"this one says: I am, I am the bulky head"

(b)

thumb	*äni båt bašin duzdi*	"this one said: let's go thieving"
foref.	*äni båt kuǰå bašin*	"this one said: where shall we go?"
middle f.	*äni båt šåhi kia*	"this one said: to the King's house"
ring f.	*äni båt a meniun*	"this one said : I am not coming"

---

ferent linguistic levels (highly standardized in the case of European languages, such as French, Italian, English, etc.).

22 An appendix with different types of finger rhymes in German languages is given in BENNETT 1982: 18–21; see also ERDAL 1981: 124–125. A couple of rhymes in Maghrebine Arabic are in CHEBEL 1999: 89. A few examples from Italian folklore are in ALINEI 2009: 271–272.

little f.	*äni båt kulla, kulla šämširka* *därun.mukun, mäšin, mukun, miun*	"this one said: I am a big, big little sword. I strike and go, I strike and come"

A short Xuri finger rhyme, very close to a rhyme I used to patter when I was a child, sounds as follows (ŠĀYEGĀN 2006: 171):

little f.	*emmorγu sareow*	"this small bird is near the water"
ring f.	*em begeraftē*	"this one seized it"
middle f.	*em bekoštē*	"this one killed it"
foref.	*em bepedē*	"this one cooked it"
thumb	*em befārdē*	"this one ate it"

The mere fact that each finger is reckoned as different from the others and endowed with an individual personality is a current motif in many Ir. proverbs. In the following Prs. proverbs, the differences among fingers symbolize the differences among human people:

> *angošt-e kučak folān nemitavānad šod*
> "the little finger cannot become any Tom, Dick and Harry";[23]
> *panǰ angošt barādar and, barābar nistand*
> "the five fingers are brothers, not equal";
> *panǰ angošt yeki nistand*[24]
> "the five fingers are not one and the same";
> *xodā panǰ angošt rā yek andāze nayāfaride*
> "God did not create the five fingers of the same size";
> *xodā dah angošt rā barābar xalq nakarde*
> "God did not create the ten fingers equal".[25]

These Prs. proverbs find parallels in both Iranian and not Iranian traditions; cf. Pšt. *pin<u>dz</u>ah wáṛah gute barábare nah dí* "all five fingers are not alike (= all men are not alike)" (GILBERTSON 1932: s.v. *finger*); Ar. (variety

[23] One may resort to this proverb to stress that "there is no equal to a so-and-so in doing something" (DEHX).

[24] A Zarq. (Fārs) version (*panš tā angošt mesle ham nis*) is in MALEKZĀDE 2004: 81; an analogous Sang. proverb (*panǰ angošt kə mači nabunən* "the five fingers are not of the same size") is in TAᶜDĀDI SANGESARI 2002: 86.

[25] See ŠĀMLU 2000: 1007–1008.

spoken in the Persian Gulf area) *ṣuwwabiᶜ yaddak muub waḥda* "your fingers are not the same" (QAFISHEH 1997: s.v. *ṣubiᶜ*).[26]

There is a plenty of references to fingers in general, and specific fingers in particular, in the idiomatic phraseology of any Ir. languages. From them, one may infer the place these body parts have in the human imagery. I will not dwell upon them; I would only mention the Prs. expression *šast-e kasi xabardār šodan* (lit. 'to become aware, said of someone's thumb'), which means 'to find out suddenly; to perceive, understand by instinct' (NAJAFI 1999),[27] and presupposes the identification of the thumb, a perceptive antenna, with the whole person. The "alert thumb" strongly reminds the Shakespearean "pricking thumbs" ("By the pricking of my thumbs – something wicked this way comes", *Macbeth* Act 4, Scene 1, 44–45), which has also inspired the title (*By the pricking of my thumbs*) of a famous novel by Agatha Christie.

The attitude of people towards their fingers has encouraged in many languages denomination processes based on the conceptual equation FINGER = HUMAN BEING.[28] Old Turkish *ärnäk* 'little man' (ERDAL 1981: 124), used as the general term for 'finger', is explained in the light of an anthropomorphic perspective. Being equated to human beings, fingers may also be linked each other by kindred relationships, as human beings are; this conceptual association explains many finger names, with a worldwide, albeit discontinuous, distribution.

7. The lexical domain of the finger names shows astonishing analogies in the conceptual grounds from which it has developed in the different languages, analogies which may be explained resorting to the common experi-

---

26 Something similar should exist in Gypsy folklore as well. As reported by an Italian journalist interviewing a young Romani woman after several acts of aggression against Rom camps in a few Italian cities, planned in reprisal of criminal acts allegedly committed by Romani people, the woman stated that the collective punishment was to be considered as unjust, since Romanies are different one from the other, and she accompanied her wording with the moving of the fingers of one of her hands.

27 Similarly, cf. Sang. *ma šast xabar dār bəbo* (TaᶜDĀDI SANGESARI 2002: 143) and Neh. *šasseš âmu xabar*, with which one remarks the fact that a piece of news has been spread earlier than one could image (SOTUDE 1989: 75).

28 Among the different parts composing the human body, however, not only the fingers can be perceptually conceived as human beings. On the anthropomorphic and, in general, animistic patterns in the development of the body part terminology see also BONFANTE 1958.

ence of mankind and to the perceptive and cognitive abilities shared by human beings.

The finger names derive from cognitive processes in which the fingers are described in terms of some peculiar features or are equated with something different on the basis of associative principles. We can distinguish three main tendencies: the emphasis may be laid (1) on the physical appearance of the fingers; (2) on their relative position; (3) on one of the possible (real or symbolic) functions or activities people commonly assign to them.

Fingers' appearance and position represent anatomic universals based on a common perceptual reality. This does not mean however that all the people all over the world would describe their fingers in the same way. Starting from one and the same reality, different aspects may be selected and intervene in the denomination processes.

The thumb may be perceived as a big or as a short finger, depending on the touchstone. Its dimension and shape may favour mental processes based on associative principles which equate the finger to another element belonging to a different domain. The equation may be dependent on sociocultural constraints. It is a matter of fact that, from an anatomical point of view, all people the world over have any of their fingers at the same position with respect to the others. But one may decide, for example, to describe the position of the ring finger with respect to the middle finger or with respect to the little finger. Fingers may also be examined in their sequential order. But when people use their fingers in counting, the finger from which computation starts may differ according to different cultural practices: there are people starting from their thumb, others from their little finger, and there are those who, by cutting off the thumb, start the sequence from their forefinger. In the Middle East, computation generally starts with the little finger.[29] This current practice has originated a few Ar. expressions, with which one may emphasise the importance attributed to the person one is talking about. When equating a person to a bent little finger, the first to be counted, the speaker acknowledges him/her as 'the first', the top in his/her category (see LANE 1968: s.v. *xinṣir* and *ṯhanna*). The finger names which take into account the finger sequential position clearly show the culturally imposed order. In English, for example, the forefinger, *alias* the first finger, is obviously considered to be the first. This order is proved to be very common in

29 ŠĀYEGĀN (2006: 171) remarks the fact that Xuri children always begin counting with their little finger.

different areas of the world.[30] However, even in English one may note pattern stratifications: if *first finger* may only refer to the forefinger (never the thumb!), and consequently *second finger* is used with reference to the middle finger, *third finger* to the ring finger and *fourth finger* to the little finger, it sometimes happens to find the expressions *third finger* and *fourth finger* in connection with the middle finger and the little finger, respectively.[31]

Names for fingers motivated by activities performed by, or attributed to fingers are generally culturally bounded. However, functional universals also exist. This is proved by several iconomastic types for finger names pointing to specific activities, which are shared by people from different cultural backgrounds and speaking different languages, as is the case with "the pointing finger" and "the plate licking finger" for the forefinger or "the lice squatting finger" for the thumb.

8. Not all the languages have specific names for all the fingers. In some languages, only the thumb and the little finger have their own denominations, with the other ones having no name or being referred to with a general term for 'finger' (taxonomic subordination change). Different factors may favour this situation. Even alleged magic powers could suggest not giving a name, as could be the case with the ring finger.

However, when a specific finger is simply recorded with the general term for 'finger', one has to be cautious. Much may depend on how the data has been recorded. Specific elicitation techniques, for instance, may guide the informant towards a particular kind of answer, with the danger of distortions. Suppose an informant, inquired after the name of a single finger, is not in the position to answer the question, since he fails a specific name, being missing in his dialectal repertoire (what is likely) or in his personal, active repertoire (what is more likely). On this specific occasion, he may follow different strategies. He may say, for example, that he does not know it; he may say that that finger does not have any name at all, or he may get out of the tight corner resorting to the general (categorically superordinate) term for 'finger'. In a section dedicated to 'Sentences relating to parts of the body' in a Balochi handbook first published in the 1960s (ᶜABDULQAYYŪM BALOČ 1997: 198), we read that «*mardume dastā panč lankuk int. awli zandê māsī ā diga-*

30 For Dravidian, for example, cf. Parji *muna vanda* DED² 5020 'the finger which is ahead'.

31 See for instance the definition of Engl. *finger* in COD: «One of the five terminal members of hand (*thumb, & index, middle, ring, & little*, ff.), or four excluding thumb (usu. now membered thus, but cf. *fourth f.*, i.e. *ring f.*, in marriage service)».

rān lankuk gušant» (“In the hand of a man there are five fingers [*lankuk*]. The first, stout one is called *māsī*, the other ones are called *lankuk* [‘finger’]”). It is in this light that we should probably interpret the data provided by ŽUKOVSKIJ (1888: 63) for Kešei, where *aŋguš* should be ‘finger’ but also ‘forefinger’, ‘middle finger’, and ‘ring finger’, or for Vonišuni (ibid.), where *uŋguss* stands for ‘finger’, ‘forefinger’, ‘middle finger’, ‘ring finger’ and ‘little finger’.

The following anecdote is clear and to the point. Pressed by Grace Goodell, a young American researcher working in a village of Xuzestān on the bird lore and trying to straighten out some of the village bird names and descriptions, the sage Old Nur, a 87-year-old man living in Rahmat-Ābād, spoke in this way: «“Sometimes Long Tail wants to sing this way, sometimes another tune ! […] Call all the little ones sparrows, Khanom Grace; write down that the big ones are named hawks.” He held up his hand, opened out. “One finger is long, one is short, one is fat,” he said; “they’re all different. Some of us are Lurs, some Arabs, Bakhtiaris, some mahalli, one American. Hosein is dark, Fatemeh is blond, Abol has green eyes. […] Everything’s different, individual, each has its own job, that’s all. This finger points, these two pick up bread, this one wears a ring, this one is too small to do anything. Call these all fingers, call all the birds sparrows. What does it matter? Call all the big ones hawks, all the little ones sparrows. Who can begin to name every little bone and muscle of God’s hand?”» (GOODELL 1979: 152).

CHAPTER TWO: THE FINGER

0. This chapter will deal with the Ir. words for 'finger', grouped according to their iconomastic type, and inside these groupings, according to their etymons.

Historical linguists classify FINGER among the concepts for which no 'common' IE word did exist. Iconymastic regularities suggest that words for 'finger' in IE languages had in most cases CROOKEDNESS, POINTEDNESS, EXTREMITY, etc. as their original concept sources.[32] This means that the shape of the finger represents the most predictable motivation for its designation.

In Iranian, several terms for 'finger' are connected to the concepts of CROOKEDNESS (§ 1) or STRAIGHTNESS (§ 2). The finger's shape is responsible for a recurrent associative pattern that equates this part of the body with a reed, a shoot, a thorn or other small and straight things, belonging to the botanic domain. Several figurative expressions have been produced in this way, whose transparency, however, has in most cases gone lost (§ 3).

The collocation of the fingers in the human body frame is a salient feature, which has favoured the recourse to conceptual associations based on contiguity (and in a few cases metaphorical mapping), with the semantic extension to 'finger' of terms originally referring to 'five fingers / hand', 'knuckle joint', 'nail', 'paw', etc. (§ 4).

Few Ir. terms for 'finger' result from a conceptualization process where SMALLNESS appears to be the source concept (§ 5). Some might be explained as the result of the metaphorical mapping FINGERS = HUMAN BEINGS, with a kindred relationship attributed to them (§ 6).

Terms for 'finger' evoking one of the many functions people attribute to this part of the body are very few in Iranian (§ 7). Borrowings from non-Ir. languages are not rare (§ 8).

Retracing the iconym underlying each term proved to be a difficult task. Many of the proposals advanced in this chapter are to be considered as mere conjectures; a number of problems in interpretation (both on etymological and iconological bases) still remain to be solved. Isolated terms, which I was not able to classify, are collected at the end of this chapter (§ 9).

---

32 Cf. BUCK 1949: 239–240; BONFANTE 1939: 206–207.

1.1. To the notion of CROOKEDNESS point Prs. *angošt* 'finger' and its several cognates, attested in Old- (Av. *angušta-*), Middle- (MPrs. *angust/št*, Man. Prth. *angušt*, Sgd. *angušt*, Khot. *haṃguṣṭa-*[33]) and New Iranian. They are commonly referred to the IE base **ank/g-* 'to bend' (IEW 45–46); as for the *-st-* suffixation (cf. e.g. **pn̥kʷsti-* > Engl. *fist*), which «appears in other words pertaining to the hand and its parts», see SCHWARTZ 1992: 424.

Prs. *angošt* and cognates have their IA counterparts; here belongs Skt. *aṅguṣṭhá-* 'thumb, big toe' with its modern outcomes (cf. EWA I: 49, CDIAL 137).

In Avestan, *angušta-* is not the usual word for 'finger' (see below, § 2). Taking into consideration its actual attestations (BARTHOLOMAE 1904), scholars argued that Av. *angušta-* would convey the meaning 'finger' only in compounds; otherwise it would mean 'toe'. One would be led to conclude that Av. *angušta-* has undergone a semantic change, reducing its range to the specialized sense of 'toe', with the old sense 'finger' still preserved in frozen compounds.[34] This is also what MAYRHOFER assumes, when in EWA I, s.v. *aṅguṣṭhá-* 'Daumen', he quotes Av. *angušta-* 'Zehe'. The scanty occurrences of this word in the Avestan corpus do not allow to confirm that *angušta-* means specifically 'toe'. On the contrary, the relevant passages in which it means unequivocally 'toe' (four times in *Vd.* 8.70–71), where the reference to the body lower limbs is beyond discussion, induce to think that Av. *angušta-* simply means 'digit', just as MPrs. *angušt,* Prs. *angošt*, etc. do.

The following list shows the large diffusion of the *angošt*-type forms in modern Iranian:

Prs. *angošt,* Taj. *angušt*, Badaxš. *angüšt*, Madagl. *angüšt*, Tāti (Apšeron) *œngÿšt* (GRJUNBERG 1963: 117), Birǰ. *ongoš(t)*, Qāi. *ɛngoš*, TrbHayd. *angušt*, Šir. *angošt*, Esf.Prs. *angoš(d)*, Šušt. *angos*, Ham. *engošt*, *ongušt*, Bxt. *angust* (LORIMER 1922), *angušt* (VAHMAN – ASATRIAN 1987), Lo. (Bālā-Gar.) *añušt,* Mamas. *aŋgɔšt* (ANONBY 2003: 186), Zarq. *angošt*, Bast. *āngošt*, Lār. *angošt*;

SulKrd. *emust,* SouthKrd. *angus(t), amust*, Krmnš. *angušt,* Sin. *angᴜs*, Gor. *angušt*, Awr. *angᴜsa,* Zā. *engişt* (TODD 1985), (Çermik-Siverek and Palu-Bingöl) *gišt* (PAUL 1998);[35]

---

33 Also spelt *hagauṣṭa*; cf. BAILEY 1979: 442a and 439b.

34 In fact, as R. SCHMITT has kindly pointed out to me, only an Av. compound containing *angušta-* is attested (*darəyō-angušta- Yt.* 17.11).

35 See also below, p. 86.

Āmor. *ešgonda* (ᶜĀDELXĀNI 2000), *ongošta* (MOQDAM 1949: 33),[36] Kah. *engošt*, Āšt. *engošt*, Vfs. *æengosde* (*æengoste* MOQDAM 1949: 33), Biz. *angöš*, Yzd. *æengošt*, Kāšāni *unguss*, Mah. *uñgušt*, Ardest. *engušt*, Del. *angošda, ayngošdae*, Ār.-Bidg. *əgüš*, Esf-JPrs *ongoθ*, Xuns. *ongoss*, Xur. *āngos*, Abiā. *angöšt*, Siv. *gūs* (LECOQ 1979 *gos*),[37] Kerm., ZorKerm. *engošt*, Nāi. *engošt* (besides *engoli*) (LECOQ 2002), Farizandi *aŋgošt*, Keš. *aŋguš* (*aŋgušt* KRAHNKE 1976: 227), Mei. *ɔngošt*, Nohuǰi *ɛngʋst*, Qohr. *enüšt* (*angüšt*), Soi *ängüšt*, Gz. *engušt*, Voniš. *uŋguss*, Bohr. *eŋgüš*, Abd. *angušt* (ŽUKOVSKIJ 1922: 110), Sed. *uŋguss*, Tarqi *aŋgʋst*, Yarandi *aŋgošt*, Nat. *äŋgošt, oŋgošt* (CHRISTENSEN 1930: 289);[38]

Māz. (West.) *angis*, (East.) *angus,* (ᶜAli Ābād) *angust* (SOTUDE 1962), IrĀz. *āngišt* (KĀRENG 1954), (Ešt.) *angušta* (YARSHATER 1969: 58), (Sagz.) *angušte*, (Ebr., Xoi.) *angušta*, (Čā.) *anguš(t)a*, (Harz.) *ungüšt*, Gil. *angušt*, Tāl. *angušta*, (Māsule) *angišt* (LAZARD 1979), (Māsāl) *angušta* (NAWATA 1982: 108), Srx. *engošt*, Semn. *angošt(a)*, Šahm. *angošt*, Sang. *angošt*, Lāsg. *engošt*, Aft. *engošt*, Qasr. *angušd*;

Pšt. *gúta, gwə́ta, angúšt* (< Prs.), Wan. *nəgút , nogút,* Dzadr. *gwə́ta*, Yγn. *angúšt*, Ōrm. *aŋguṣ̌t,* (MORGENSTIERNE 1932b) *nᵘŋgušt*, Par. *aŋgušt, γošt* (*γušt* IIFL-I),[39] Sgl. *iŋgī̆t*, Išk. *ingit* (*iŋgiṭ* IIFL-II), Ydγ. *oguščo*, Mnǰ. *agūšḱa* (*āguškyo* IIFL-II), Šγn. *angix̌t*, Bart., Xuf., Oroš., Roš., Baǰ. *ingax̌t* (EVŠG), Yzγ. *γʷax̌t,* Sariq. *i/ïngax̌t, i/ůngax̌t*, etc.

As it clearly appears at first glance, cognates of Prs. *angošt* are widespread almost everywhere in Iranian, though not in a uniform way. In Kurdish, the *angošt*-forms differentiate Central and Southern Kurdish, where they are actually used, from Northern Kurdish, where they are not.[40] The common Bal. word for ‘finger’ is not an *angošt*-type one, even if Bal. speakers from

---

36 The two sources differ (the former giving a form with metathesis). A derivative of this word is Āmor. *angošdak* ‘tonsils’ (ADIB TUSI 1963–1964).

37 For Siv. *gos* ‘index finger’ see below, p. 131.

38 A good collection of *angošt*-type forms in the Central dialects is in KRAHNKE 1976: 227.

39 MORGENSTIERNE (IIFL I: 257 f.) points to the same etymological connection, though, he adds, «Av. *vītasti-* “span” would also have resulted in Par. **γušt*».

40 KURDOEV 1960 marks *engûşt* as “Southern Kurdish”; AMÎRXAN 1992 gives *embust* as meaning ‘Fingerbreite; Spannweite zwischen Daumen und Mittelfinger’. Cf. however *emust* ‘Finger’ in OMAR 1992.

the Lāšār (Iran) and Kang (Afghanistan) areas[41] do say *angušt* for 'finger', taking it directly from (Afγ)Persian. I found no confirmation of Bal. *gutā* (or *gut* + obl. marker?), recorded in the sentence *anguštrī āī-gutā diyant* ("they put a ring on his finger") and reported as Balochi Makrāni in GRIERSON 1921: 381. This form has also been quoted by MORGENSTIERNE in EVP s.v. *gūta* («lw? But also Bal. *īt* 'brick', *phut* 'back' with *t* < *št*»). Moreover, one should always consider that some forms which do exist in a given language, and are recorded by lexicographers, may be not central in the lexicon of that language, or may be restricted to specific linguistic registers, while other words, sometimes not recorded by lexicographers, may be preferred in everyday life. According to PURHOSEYNI (1991), for instance, Prs. speakers of Kermān preferably call the finger *nāxun* (see below, p. 84) rather than *angošt*, which PURHOSEYNI also records in his Kerm. dictionary.

Without entering into the merits of the complicated problem of an adequate selection of distinctive features for a new classification of Western Iranian, I would like to draw attention to the well known phenomenon of palatalization loss in the cluster *-št-* (no. 14 in TEDESCO 1921, illustrated with the couple *rāšt* : *rāst*), generally taken as a Persian, and then SWIr., feature. Though in more recent approaches to Ir. dialectology (see LECOQ 1989b or WINDFUHR 1995) this trait is no more taken into consideration, Prs. *angošt* still continues to be quoted as a "NWIr. lw.". From the *angošt*-list provided above, it clearly emerges that the *-st-* forms (both with cluster maintained, and reduction of the cluster with loss of the final dental) are not a peculiarity of the so-called Southern varieties, as one would expect it: they occur in Kurdish and Gorāni, in a few Central dialects and in Māzandarāni. Inside the Persic group, only Baxtiāri has both *-st-* and *-št-* forms, just as Middle Persian had.

From the **ang*-base to which Prs. *angošt* belongs, several Ir. words pertaining to the anatomical domain derive. See Khot. *aṃga-* 'limb', Lir.-Dayl. *ang* 'finger joint' (LIRĀVI 2001: 217), to which, for IA, Skt. *aṅgá-* 'body limb' (EWA, I: 48) may be added.

Derivatives (with or without prothetic *h-*) and connected forms are: Khot. *haṃgari* 'part of the body', EBal. *angwā(h)* 'limb, member' (MIṬHĀ – SURAT 1970), Birǰ. *engam* 'limb', IrĀz. (Xoi.) *angela* 'arm', (Čā.) *angala* 'sleeve' (YARSHATER 1969: 35), Tafr. *angīna* 'elbow' (ADIB TUSI 1963–

41 See also *angušt* in ELFENBEIN 1990-I: 45 (20), in a poem written by Nūr Muhammad Bāmpuštī (the district of Bāmpušt is located southwest of Sarāwān, in Persian Balochistan).

1964), Krd. (Mahâb.) *hangil̠* 'armpit', Lo. *hangel* 'armpit, shoulder', (Bālā-Gar.) *hañal* 'armpit', Naqusāni *angila* 'sleeve' (DARUDIĀN 1986), etc. A detailed discussion of this lexical group is postponed to another occasion. What concerns us for now is that here also belong the words that will be treated in the next paragraph.

1.2. Prs. *angol* (with *angolak, angulak*) derives from **ang-*, just as *angošt* does.[42] It does not mean 'finger', not, at least, in the current Prs. use, though FF gives it simply as 'finger [*angošt, asba*ᶜ]'. It rather means 'a slight touch with the finger' (HAIM 1992a, ĀRYĀNPUR KĀŠĀNI 1979, etc.), that kind of touch which may produce 'excitation, chatouillement' (LAZARD 1990a s.v. *angolak*). To put it briefly, nowadays *angol* is used in Persian with the meaning of 'fingering', i.e. (1) handling or touching with the fingers in many senses, but generally with a slight negative implication (*angošt zadan*) or (2) putting one's finger into (*angošt kardan*), like to put finger into one's nose, into one's mouth, etc. To this latter sense is related an obscene sense ('to stuff the finger up the bottom'), current in Persian (mainly with *angolak*) and in many other Ir. languages and mostly recorded in the relevant dictionaries.

It is however reasonable to think that the original meaning of this Prs. *l*-derivative form was 'finger'; it is surely 'finger' in a 12th c. text, the *Mujmal al-tawārīx*, whose author was probably native to the region of Hamadān (LAZARD 1963: 119). There, Ardašēr is depicted as being *dirāz-angul* ('long fingered').[43] It still retains the meaning 'finger' in Fārs: cf. Dav. *angol,* Sarv. *angol*, Kāz. *angol*, etc. BEHRUZI (1969) attributes two senses to Šir. *angol*: (1) 'finger', and (2) 'finger when inserted somewhere, like into the nose, etc.'. For the Baxtiāri area, ANONBY (2003: 187) gives ČLang *aŋgoli*;[44] moving southwards one finds Buš. *angol* and Lir-Dil. *angûl*. Birǰ. *angol* '(1) finger; (2) to put one's finger into someone's bottom' has been recorded in the Birǰ. glossary of Mollā ᶜAli Ašraf Sabuhi (19th c.) and is probably out of date; nowadays Birǰ. speakers currently use *ongoš*(*t*) 'finger'. In Sistāni and Minābi, *angol* is the name of the middle finger; on the common conceptual shift FINGER → MIDDLE FINGER, see below, p. 140.

---

42 For Skt. *aṅgúri-, aṅgúli-* 'finger, toe' and its several IA cognates see EWA I: 49 and CDIAL 135.

43 See quotation in DEHX, s.v. As R. SCHMITT has kindly pointed out to me, the expression *dirāz angul* referred to *Ardašēr* (*Artaxerxes*) could also be an equivalent of *dirāz dast* (*Longimanus*).

44 According to SARLAK (2002), the word for 'finger' in ČLang Bxt. is *kelek*; see below, p. 63.

To find a more compact diffusion of *l*-derivatives from *ang*-forms, we have to look at the Central dialects. KRAHNKE (1976: 227–228 and Map V – 33) has demonstrated how the diffusion of these forms reinforces the northern/southern differentiation inside the whole Central area investigated by the author, already outlined by other isoglosses. A homogeneous presence of the *angol*-type characterizes the southern part, while the northern is mostly characterized by the *angošt*-type.

One may quote Nāi. *engoli,* Anār. *engili*, Varz. *angoli*, Gz. *ĕŋgolī, ĕŋgulī*, Kuhp. *eŋgulī,* Kāšāni *engulī* (MORGENSTIERNE 1932a: 40), ZorKerm./Yzd. *angol*, Sed. *uŋgulī,* Kafr. *eŋgulī*, Zefr. *üŋgülī*, Nat. *eŋgulī*, Abčuyei *aŋguli* (KRAHNKE 1976: 227), etc.

To these forms, one should add Esf.Prs. *anguli* recorded as 'finger' and 'to finger' in DĀDMĀN 1976.

Isolated *l*-forms are found here and there in different dialectal areas, cf. Māz. *engel*, quoted by MORGENSTIERNE 1932a: 40, with most probability taken from CHODŹKO 1842: 581.[45] ELFENBEIN 1990-II[46] cites Bal. *angul* (seemingly taking it from MORGENSTIERNE ibid.; Noške), a form for which I found no confirmation in my interviews with Bal. speakers native to different dialectal areas. It is quite possible, however, that *angul* is (was?) used somewhere in Balochistan (under IA influence? cf. Khetr. *aŋʌl*, Sir. *aṅgal*).[47] From a Bal. speaker from Nasirābād I recorded *angrī, angurī* 'finger', a clear IA loanword, possibly related to Si. *āguri*.

In EIr., *l*-forms for 'finger' are Oss. *ængwylʒ* (Dig. *ængulʒæ*) and Wx. *yanglək, yangl*: see respectively IESOJ and STEBLIN-KAMENSKIJ 1999 SV., with etymological references.

2. The common Av. term for 'finger' (and 'toe') is *ərəzu-*, a word for which only an isolated correspondence in the Oss. anatomical lexicon (Oss. *wyrz,* Dig. *urz* 'finger-tip') has been suggested so far.[48] The identification of

---

45 CHODŹKO quotes Māz. *engel* 'finger' commenting the line *še keše engeli kude*. At page 581 we read: «*engeli* from انكل "a finger, (whence *enghel*, a ring)," literally, this word means "the scratching with fingers"». I found no attestation of this word in the Māz. dictionaries at my disposal.

46 However, it does not occur in any of the texts of the *Anthology*.

47 That Bal. *angul* could be considered as a lw. from IA has been questioned by MORGENSTIERNE (1932a: 40) and KORN (2005: 293).

48 STEBLIN-KAMENSKIJ (1999: 459 s.v. Wx. *wʋrzg(ə)* 'right (of hand)') connects some EIr. words for 'right' (see already IIFL II: 192) with Av. *ərəzu-* "straight, right" (BARTHOLOMAE 1904 [1]*ərəzu-*), without further comments.

the salient feature of this body part responsible for this Av. denomination is debated. The hypothesis most frequently quoted in the literature (BARTHOLOMAE 1904, IEW, BUCK 1949: 40, etc.) rests on the ability of fingers to stay upright: Av. *ərəzu-* (YAv. [3]*ərəzav-* in BARTHOLOMAE 1904) would be a nominalization of the adjective *ərəzu-*, attested in Gathic with the meaning of 'gerade, richtig, recht' ([1]*ərəzav-* in BARTHOLOMAE 1904), and would consequently belong to IE **reĝ-* 'straight' (IEW 854). This derivation has been strongly challenged by ABAEV (IESOJ s.v. *wyrz*): according to him, peculiar features of a finger are mobility and disposition to bend, and not capacity to be straight. ABAEV suggests a derivation from an IE base **u̯er-ĝh- / u̯renĝh-* 'to turn' (IEW 1154–1155); according to his proposal, the Av. term for 'finger' would evoke one of the many actions commonly performed by the fingers, which would be prototypically perceived as "claspers", and would join the other Ir. words for 'finger' which find their motivation in specific functions attributed to fingers (§ 7). The quasi-isolation of Av. *ərəzu-* 'finger' inside Iranian makes it more difficult to take a stand and to accept one hypothesis rather than another, and it is also possible that ABAEV is right in rejecting the previous proposal.[49] What could be contested to ABAEV on the semantic level, however, is the reason of his refusal: if it is true that the fingers are highly flexible elements, it is just as true that they can be kept straight; in fact, many of the "actions" performed by the fingers are realized by straightening one or more fingers.

3. The shape the fingers assume when they are kept straight have favoured the creation of words for 'finger' which equate them to reeds, sprouts, branches, etc. However, the direction of the metaphorical association may also be inverted; clear instances are Taj. *panǰa* 'leaf; branch', IrĀz. *penǰa* 'blade of grass poking up from the ground' (ADIB TUSI 1963–1964), etc.[50]

Among the motivations underlying words for 'finger', this is one of the most privileged. Fingers depicted as twigs, boughs, etc. are also found in Sanskrit; see for example *karaśākhā-* 'finger' (< *kará-* 'hand' + *śākhā-* 'branch'; Lex., CDIAL 2801), *kará-pallava-* 'finger' (< *kará-* + *pallava-* 'sprout, twig'; CDIAL 7969), *śáryā-* 'cane, shaft, arrow; finger', *śalākā-*

[49] ABAEV's etymological suggestion for Av. *ərəzu-* is considered untenable by R. SCHMITT (p.c.): to accept it, one should admit an unjustified loss of initial **v-*.

[50] On the *panǰe*-type words for 'finger' (FIVE → FIVE FINGERS → FINGER) see § 4.1 below.

'any small stake or stick; finger', etc. Evidence of the presence of this iconomastic type in Iranian will be produced in what follows.[51]

3.1. Although *angušt* is well established in literary Tajik, speakers of several Taj. dialects prefer using other labels for 'finger'. In South-East Tajikistan (Kara-Tegin and Darvāz), they use *lik,* in Badaxšān and Vanǰ, *likak, likək* (ROZENFEL'D 1982); cf. also Badaxš. *lakük, likīk,* Madagl. *lakīk* in LORIMER 1922. Here possibly belongs the Bal. general term for 'finger', *lankuk* (variants: Noške *lunkuk,* Sarāwān *lankutk,* Mirǰāve (COLETTI 1981) *langotk,* SBal. (SAYAD HASHMI 2000) *lakkuk*), spread all over Western and Southern Balochi,[52] in connection of which MORGENSTIERNE (1932a: 40) mentions Gypsy Prs. *lekik* and Kumz. *linkit*. ELFENBEIN (1992: 252) submits a different explanation: *lankuk* «must ultimately belong» to *angul*, «through some form such as **lankul*».[53]

Dial. Taj. *likak*, Gypsy Prs. *lekik,* Kumz. *linkit* and Bal. *lankuk* might be somehow connected with a set of adjectives, meaning 'straight, erect, upright', among which there are AfγPrs. *lek, leq*, Birǰ. *lek*, Sist. *lakk*, SBal. *lik*,[54] Pšt. (also Dzadr.) *lak* ('stiff, standing, rigid, unbending'). Here might also belong Pšt. *lakáy* 'tail of animal or bird', Ōrm. *likiē* 'tail' (MORGENSTIERNE 1932b), and probably Haz. *lak* 'erection, membrum virile' (DULLING 1973).

The *lek*-'straight' adjectival set, mostly spread in the Iranian East, could be associated to another lexical set, more compactly diffused in the Iranian West (particularly in Kurdish, Gorāni and Lori), including words meaning

---

51 Possibly, one has to interpret in this perspective the Prs. expression *qolzom-e panǰ-šāx* 'palm of the hand and the fingers of a munificent man' (FF).

52 The current EBal.word for 'finger' is *murdān*(*ag*); see below, § 7.1.

53 STEBLIN-KAMENSKIJ agrees on this point, as stated by ELFENBEIN.

54 SAYAD HASHMI 2000. The real diffusion of Bal. *lik(k)* inside SBal. escapes me. SAYAD HASHMI 2000 mostly provides Makrāni/Coastal lexicon, but with many inconsistencies. MAYER (1910, s.v. *to erect*) marks *lik kanaga* as "South Balochi". Cf. also *lik kanaga* 'to erect, to cause to stand' in PIERCE 1875. An occurrence of *likk* is found in ELFENBEIN 1983a: 24(20), in a version of the well known story of Leyla and Maǰnun (*yak roče ātk yak dārburre, dīt-ī ki yak dāre lik-in* "one day a woodcutter came, he saw that a tree-trunk is standing"); the dialect of the ms. should be a Coastal one, as also assumed by ELFENBEIN (ibid.: 3). Bal. *likk* is also present in AYYUBI 2002 (SBal. of Iran, *lekk* 'erect, firm'). A Bal. speaker from Turbat (Pakistani Makrān) told me that he does not use *likk* in this sense; however, he provided me with the derivative *likkū* 'on tiptoe'. On the other hand, the verbal compound *likk kapag* 'to climb' is well known and used everywhere in Balochi.

'shooting, bough, twig'[55] or the like. These are: KurmKrd. *liq* (RIZGAR 1993), Sul. *lik, liq*, SouthKrd. *leq, liq, lik, like*, (Mahâb.) *lik, liq*, (Garr.) *läq e dâr* 'branch', Lak. *l̆ik* ('sprout'), Gor. (Kand.) *läq*, Bxt. *lek* (see also *lik* 'ear of corn' in LORIMER 1922),[56] *lak* 'shoot, twig, blade of grass' (LORIMER 1955: 100), Mamas. *lighghä* 'Baumast', *laghä* 'Ast' (MANN 1910), Gavk. *laɣa* 'branch', Dav., Dahl., Knd., Mās. *lâɣa*, Kāz., Kuz. *lâɣe* 'bough' (SALĀMI 2004: 126–127), Tāl. *lok* 'petite branche' (MILLER 1930), etc.

3.2. The mental association (PART OF) FINGER = REED probably motivates a group of Ir. words used as general terms for 'finger', which may be related to Prs. *kelk* 'hollow reed' (a "rare" word in Prs., according to LAZARD 1990a). Such a connection has already been suggested by different scholars, among which MONCHI-ZADEH (1990: 106) for Xor. *klīk* and CABOLOV (2001) for Krd. *kilk* 'finger'. Cognates of Prs. *kelk* are also used in the Ir. body lexicon as a denomination of 'tail' (mainly in Kurdish and Gorāni).

The *kelk*-type words for 'finger' are mostly found in Central and Southern Kurdish (as contrasted with Northern Kurdish, where *kilk* is 'tail'), Gorāni and Lori clusters, in Lārestāni and Eastern Persian: cf. SulKrd. *kilk*, SouthKrd. *kilk* 'finger; tail; reed', (Krmnš.) *kelek*, (Garr.) *kel̆īk*, (Sennai) *kelk* etc. (CHRISTENSEN – BARR 1939: 305–306 with further references) 'finger',[57] Lak. *kel̆ek*, Gor. (Kand.) *kilk* 'Finger', *kilikä* 'Zehe', (Gahw.) *kilik* (HADANK 1930: 259–260; see there for further references), (Talahed.) *kelek*, Arāk. *kelek*, Āvarz. *kelek*, Šušt. *kelek*, Lo. *kelek*, (Bālā-Gar.) *killik* (also 'stick'), Dezf. *kelek* (EMĀM 2000: 97), Bxt. (ČLang) *kelek*,[58] (Pāgač) *kelik*, all meaning 'finger'. In Fārs, one finds *kelek* in (Krd.) Koruni. In SE and NE Iran, the presence of the *kelk*-type 'finger' is assured by Lārest. *kelik*, Farām. *kelik* 'finger' and Xor. *kalīk*, TrbHayd. *kelik* (see also *keliki* 'finger-ring'),

---

55 I tentatively suggest correlating them with the large group of IA words, mostly meaning 'club, stock', gathered in CDIAL (10875 and Add.) s.v. *lakuṭa-*; cf. also KEWA III: 84–85; EWA II: 472.

56 The hypothesis advanced by VAHMAN – ASATRIAN (1987), connecting Bxt. *lik, lek* to Prs. *lik* 'a measure for corn or dates', seems improbable to me (unless there is some connection between the denomination of the measuring instrument and segments of reeds or the like).

57 For a dialectal differentiation of this word (*kılıg*: Kalhori of Šâhbâd, Mandili, Badra, Šerwâni, Malikšây, Xânaqin, Ilâm, Qasiri, surrounding of Sahana; *kılığ* Warmzyâr; *kılık* Kirmânšâh, Bilawar, Kordali, Bijâr) see FATTAH 2000: 862, 865, 869, 872, 875, 878, 882, 885, 888, 891, 895, 898, 902, 905.

58 According to ANONBY 2003: 187, 'finger' in ČLang Bxt. is *aŋgoli*.

respectively. AfγPrs. *kelk* (Kāb. *kelk*) entered as a loanword the Parāči lexicon; at the time when MORGENSTIERNE was writing the *Addenda and Corrigenda* to the first volume of *Indo-Iranian Frontier Languages* (1972), *kelk* turned out to be the usual word for 'finger' among the Parāči young people.

This *kelk*-group is plausibly related to another lexical set we will call conventionally *kelič*-group; however, some lexical contamination should have intervened, as it will also be suggested below, p. 170.[59] A different (in my opinion, unacceptable) etymology was advanced by EILERS (1988: 315), who analysed Krd. *kelīč* as the result of a "Kürzung" process (< *anguli-* + *ēč*), very similar to that which has generated Siv. *gūs* 'finger'.

Several dialectal variants are found in the Baxtiāri linguistic cluster. Besides the above mentioned *kelik* in the village of Pāgač and in ČLang, one may note Bxt. *kelič* (XASRAVI 1989), HafLang *kølidʒ* (ANONBY 2003: 186); see also (Lo.) Mamas. *k̂elič* 'finger', BoirAhm. *kʲilits*, Kuh Giluye *tsɛlidz* (ANONBY 2003: 186), Baliā. *k̂elič* (also 'little finger'). Isolated among the Central dialects appear Abiānei, with *kalīč* as an alternative to *angöšt* 'finger', and Bādrudi, with *koǰilu* 'finger', a variant with metathesis of the *kelič*-type.

To Bxt. *kelič*, one should connect Šir. *kelenǰ* 'finger (usually little finger)' (XADIŠ 2000),[60] Šir-JPrs. *kerenǰ*, recorded in MORGENSTIERNE 1960: 130 (where also Arazin *čelenga* 'finger' is quoted - with question mark), isle of Qešm *kelinč* 'finger' (NURBAXŠ 1990), and, proceeding eastwards along the coast, Rod. *kelenč, kolenč*, Horm., Min. *kelenǰ*,[61] Fin. *kelenč* and SBšk. (Garu) *kelenč*.[62] Add here also Bast. *kelenǰ pā* 'to tiptoe', as well as Zarq. *kelenǰak* 'cockspur'.

It is not clear whether Šir-JPrs. *kerenǰ* has something to do with Šir. *xerenǰ(āl)* 'claw', Kāz. *xerenǰ* 'nail' (BEHRUZI 2002), Fišarvi *xerenǰ* (in the idiom

---

[59] Xuns. *keliǰ* 'dry stalk of goat's thorn', Zarq. *keleng* 'twig (for fire)', Buš. *keleng, kelenge* 'branch of tree, stalk of grass', etc. prove that the *kelič*-group and the the *kelk*-group share the same transfer possibilities (body domain ↔ botanical domain).

[60] According to BEHRUZI (1969), Šir. *kelenǰ* is only 'little finger' (see also below, p. 169); according to XAZDUZ (2002: 133) it means 'finger'. That this word is also used as a general term for 'finger' is assured by the following expression: *folāni kelenǰe kučikeye man ham nemišavad* "So-and-so is not up to the standard of my little finger", where *kučike* 'little' modifies *kelenǰ* 'finger' (XADIŠ 2000).

[61] According to SKJÆRVØ (1975), Min. *kelenǰ* usually means 'nail'; on the possible conceptual shift FINGER ↔ NAIL, cf. also below, p. 84. The usage of *kelenč* as 'nail', however, is not confirmed by the data collected by BARBERA (2004), where *penǰ* is 'nail' and *kelenč* is 'finger'.

[62] This word is contained in an unpublished lexical list collected by G. BARBERA, who kindly put his material at my disposal.

xerenǰ alubeko 'give a scratch with the point of your fingers', EQTEDĀRI 1963: 75), Dav. *xerenǰ* 'claw, talon', Buš. *xerenǰ* 'to scratch'. The similarity of the forms *kelenǰ/kerenǰ* : *xerenǰ* may only be apparent and casual; it seems however likely that some blending has occurred.[63]

There are two words for 'finger' in Farāmarzi: *kelik* (mentioned above) and *kenǰel*. The latter could belong to the *kelič*-group (with a metathesis and a nasal insertion). Moving westwards along the coast, we find Buš. *kelang* 'finger'.

Both the *kelk*-group and the *kelič*-group will be reconsidered below (Chapter seven: The little finger).

3.3. Dial. Taj. *čilik* (Darvāz, Kara-Tegin: ROZENFEL'D 1982: 203)[64] and possibly Arazin *čelenga* 'finger'[65] could be associated to a bulk of Ir. words for twigs, pieces of wood, sticks, wooden chips etc., among which one may mention Sang. *čelkê*, Semn. *čelki*, Šahm. *čilekâ*, Lāsg. *čile*, Srx. *čilik* 'chopped wood; small pieces of wood', Māz. (Āmol.) *čele* 'branch', *čeli* 'thin branch', *čelekâ* 'wood chips resulting from cutting a tree with a hatchet' (with *čelke* metaphorically meaning 'small change'), Tāl. *čila* 'dry and thin branches used as a fuel' (ABDOLI 2001), Aft. *čile* 'small pieces of wood', *čelle* 'branch', Damāv. *čel* 'thorn', *čelke* 'fragment of anything', *čilak* 'small piece of dry wood'; IrĀz. (Tākest.) *čela* 'staff' (YARSHATER 1969: 58), KurmKrd. *çilak, çelak* 'thin cudgel' (*çil* 'branch; twig', *çîl* 'sprout, stalk' KURDOEV 1960; *çilo* 'branches (cut with leaves to feed animals)' RIZGAR 1993), SouthKrd. *čil, čalang* 'branch', *čîlka* (with metathesis, *čîkla*), *čîlik* 'short and thin branch of tree', (Krmnš.) *čileg* 'firewood', Sul. *chil̠* 'branch', *chîl̠ke* 'twig, kindling', Šir. *čileh* 'small pieces of wood; thin branch', Gavk. *čilak* 'dry, thin branch', Somγ. *čīläk* 'Stöckchen' (MANN 1909), Sarv. *čilœ* 'small and thin pieces of wood', etc. However, Taj. *čilik* and cognates,

---

63 Šir. *xerenǰ(āl)* etc. might share with Šir *xenǰāl* (XADIŠ 2000), *xenǰ* (XAZDUZ 2002: 229), Lār. *xenǰ* 'scratch' (ADIB TUSI 1963–1964), Fin. *xenǰ* 'nail, claw' a phonosymbolic origin. Worth noting is also Šir. *kelenǰār, kerenǰāl* 'crab' (XADIŠ 2000; see also Dašt. *kerenǰâl*), with *r/l* alternation and dissimilation, which could have something to do with our *kelenǰ/kerenǰ*.

64 See also KALBĀSI 1995 and MOSALMĀNIĀN QOBĀDIĀNI 1997: 32. Taj. *čilik* seems to be currently used in Yaγnobi as well; it appears in many sentences quoted in MIRZOZODA 2008 (both in the Yγn. examples and in their Taj. translations).

65 Arazin *čelenga* has been connected to Šir-JPrs. *kerenǰ* by MORGENSTIERNE (1960: 130); see above p. 64.

among which Prs. *čelk* 'little finger',[66] could also be explained in a different way; see below p. 89.

To (dial.) Taj. *čilik*, ORANSKIJ (1983: 123) doubtfully connects *čimčiloq* / *čimčaloq*, a word for 'finger' used in Jugi (*ǰugi*), one of the Tajik-based argots; for a different explanation see below, p. 172.

3.4. Kurm. Kurdish has two different words for 'finger': *pêçî* (see § 4.5.) and *tilî* (variants: *telî, tillî, tilîk*). One also finds *tilî* 'finger' in the Krd. dialect spoken in Jabal Sinǰār (Irāq; cf. BLAU 1975) and *til* in the dialects of Başqale and Zaxo. According to AWRANG (1969), *til* 'finger' is a Zā. word. A cognate word (or a lw.?) is also found in the Lori area: cf. Mamas. *tilu* 'finger' (ANONBY 2003: 186), to which one may add Lo. *kalak-e tīla* 'little finger' (see below, p. 171). The origin of this Krd. word is not clear. JABA – JUSTI (1879, s.v. *tilou* 'doigt') mention a few words from Ugric and Caucasian linguistic areas, which sound similar to the Krd. one. I suggest regarding it as an original figurative expression motivated by a metaphorical mapping and connecting it to a bulk of Ir. words for thorns, stalks, spikes, twigs etc., as is the case with Prs. *kelk*.

Consider the following: SouthKrd. *til* 'stalk of grass', KurmKrd. *t̠ila* 'branch', *têla* 'stock; rod; tree' (KURDOEV 1960), Lak. *til̃* 'offshoot; sapling just planted in the ground', Zā. (Çermik) *telī*, (Palu) *telu* 'thorn, bone(splinter)', Lo. *til* 'sapling just planted in the ground', (Bālā-Gar.) *tîl* 'cutting, twig', Xuns. *tila* 'shoot; young tree', Siv. *tīl* 'thorn',[67] Māz. *tali*, (Sār.) *tali*, *talu*, Šahm. *tali*, Šahr. *telu* 'thorn', Tāl. *telə* 'sapling of a fruit tree', etc. Ruhi Anārǰāni, the author of a very important document (*Resāle*) written in Ir. Āzari, which goes back to the 16th/17th c., used IrĀz. *til* 'sapling' in the metaphorical sense of 'male genital organ' (REZĀZĀDE MALEK 1973). In the Birǰandi dialect as it was spoken in the 19th c. and recorded by Mollā ᶜAli Ašraf Sabuhi, *tel* was used with the sense of 'chopped straw, sweeping'; nowadays Birǰ. *tel* means 'refuse, dross'.

---

66 See below, p. 170.

67 EILERS (1988) suggested deriving Siv. *tīl* 'Dorn' from *tīγ* [« < *tīγ* (phl. *tēγ*) + deminutivem *-al*? Np. *tīγāl* "(Tier-) Lager, Nest" ← "Dorngestrüpp"»], most probably because he was not aware of the large diffusion of the *til*-'thorn' type. HEJĀZI KENĀRI 1995 interprets Māz. *tali* as the result of an improbable composition (*ta-* [< Prs. *tiγ*, Phl. *tex*] + *-li* [< Phl. *lwtk* 'naked']).

Prs. dictionaries record *talu* 'thorn' (see DEHX for references). This word has no entry in FF, and is possibly a "dialectal" (< Māz. ?) term. In EIr., we find Pšt. *tiláy* 'shaft of arrow, stalks of corn after separating the heads'.

Bal. *tīlī* 'stalk of wheat; match of box' only belongs to the EBal. lexicon (MAYER 1910, GILBERTSON 1925, MIṬHĀ – SURAT 1970). EBal. *tīlī* has been borrowed from IA; cf. Si. *tīlī* 'a thin stalk of wheat; a match', Sir. *tílá* 'the final ends of reed of jungle grass etc.; a straw of wheat'; *tílí* '(1) the same as *tílá*, but shorter bits; (2) a match; (3) a twig held in left hand of drummer, on the bottom' and also Ur./Hi. *tīlī, tilī, tulī* 'a wooden or iron bar or wire (as of a bird-cage, etc.); the calf (of the leg)'.[68] One could add here Bal. *tiling* (MIṬHĀ – SURAT 1970), *tilkuk* (RAZZAQ – BUKSH – FARRELL 2001) 'peg, wooden pin', *tilk* 'piece of wood with pointed ends, etc.' (SAYAD HASHMI 2000), and perhaps also SBal. *ḍīl* 'small stick, reed' (RAZZAQ – BUKSH – FARRELL 2001), *ḍīl, ḍīllung* 'long and thin object, like the stalk of a plant or a reed', if the alternance *t/ṭ/d/ḍ* is convincingly explained. As metaphoric transfers into the anatomical domain, one may quote Bal. *ḍīl* '(human) body; stature of a person'; *daste ḍīl* 'forearm bone', *pāde ḍīllung* (SAYAD HASHMI 2000), *ṭīlling* (Turbat)[69] 'shin-bone'. Bal. *ḍīl* matches with Br. *ḍīl* 'body' (Bal. Pšt. Si., cf. ROSSI 1979: I81).

Bal. *ṭāl* 'branch; stalk of wheat; matchstick' and Pšt. *ṭāl* 'branch' are probably borrowed from IA, as well;[70] cf. the IA words collected in CDIAL 5546. Here might also belong Lārest. *tāl* 'limb, stature; height of a tree'. It is not clear if there is any direct etymological connection between an IIr. **tāla-/dāla*-type group and the IIr. lexical group, to which e.g. Krd. *til*, Ur./Hi. *tīlī, tilī*, etc. would belong.[71] In any case, contamination should have occurred between the outcomes of the two bases, with cross-borrowings both in and across Ir. and IA.

We may assume the existence of an areal lexical cluster crossing the borders of two or more linguistic families, referring to segments of trees/plants and metaphorically to body parts. I do not intend to dwell too much on this matter here. Suffice it to mention Oss. *tala* 'sapling; branch, etc.', which ABAEV (IESOJ) derives from Turk. *tal* (also *dal*) 'sapling; branch; stick' and

68 Br. *tīlī* 'splinter, stalk, spike' has been borrowed from Bal. or directly from an IA language; cf. ROSSI 1979: I330.

69 I recorded *ṭīlling* from a single Bal. speaker native to Turbat; this word, however, was unknown to other Bal. speakers from the same dialectal area, which I consulted in search of a confirmation.

70 Cf. NEVP, s.v.

71 Some of the IA words collected in CDIAL 5904 could also be associated here.

relates to several Caucasian words as well.[72] The documentation provided by ABAEV may be enlarged and include the Ir. and IA forms quoted above, or at least a part of them.

3.5. Besides *kilk*, *angust* and *qamk* (see above pp. 56, 63 and below p. 84), another word for 'finger' in Central and Southern Kurdish is *pil/pîlk*.[73] It seems to be the usual word for 'finger' at Suleymania. This Krd. word is not isolated in Iranian; cognates are attested elsewhere, even if discontinuously. In order to sketch out a possible lexical family, it will be useful to consider the semantic range covered by the Krd. lexical set to which *pil/pîlk* belongs.

HAŽĀR (1990) provides the following separate entries: (a) *pîlk* 'finger'; (b) *pil* 'hand; finger; thin offshoot of a tree; shinbone'; (c) *pal* 'limb (any arm and leg); wing of a bird; branch; thorn; arm (hand and arm); (d) *pîl* 'shoulder; limb (arm/leg)'; (e) *palik* 'branch'; (f) *balak* 'shinbone'; see also *sarpîl* 'shoulder', *pâwpil* 'leg from the foot to the knee'. Worth mentioning in BĀBĀN 1982 are: *paḻân, piḻân* 'bone' (s.v. *ostoxān*), *pêša-u-piḻânî badan* 'skeleton' (s.v. *askalat*). Beside *pil/pîlk* quoted above, WAHBY – EDMONDS (1966) also provide *pel* 'arm, limb, wing, branch'; see also (Sul. etc. dialects) *das-ū-pil* 'hand and fingers' in MACKENZIE 1961: 140. DARVIŠĀN (1996) gives Krmnš. *pal* 'arm; branch of a tree' and the compounds *pal-o-pâ* 'foot and heel [*pâ-o-pâšneye pâ*]', *pâw pal* 'legs [*par-o-pâ*]; effort [*dast-o-pâ*]'; *das-o-pel, das-o-peleng* 'hand [*dast-o-panǰe*]'. SAFIZĀDE (2001) mentions *pil* 'finger', but also 'little finger', *pêl* 'shoulder', *pal* (Gor. 'wing of bird') 'arm, arm from the elbow to the shoulder; piece; limb; body part'. For Kurmancî, CHYET 2003 provides *pîl* (also *pil*) 'arm (from shoulder to wrist); shoulder, shoulder blade', *pî* 'shoulder blade'; KURDOEV 1960 has *pel* 'shank/leg', *pîl* 'shoulder blade; arm (from shoulder to wrist)'; RIZGAR 1993 has *pîl, pî* 'shoulder blade'. However, *pîl* 'shoulder blade' may belong to another lexical group, which I will deal with elsewhere, and should be detached from here.

If one analyses all the senses recorded by the different Krd. dictionaries for the forms quoted above, one may easily recognize a conceptual homogeneity: they refer to spindle-shaped objects like young branches, etc., which

---

[72] As far as Khot. *ttīla-* ('tree, shrub' in BAILEY 1979, quoted in IESOJ) is concerned, it has been convincingly demonstrated that it is «merely the expected Prakritic form of Sanskrit *taila* 'oil'» (EMMERICK 1982).

[73] SAFIZĀDE 2001 labels *pîlk* 'finger' as "Kurmānǰi"; however, the documentation at my disposal does not confirm it.

may be equated to the human upper and lower limbs: the arm, the hand, the finger, the leg.

Outside the Kurdish area, we find the following words: Lo. *pal* 'ear of corn, branch of tree', Xuns. *pelāra* 'vine shoot', Box. *palang* 'young, small twigs of a tree' (ŠĀLČI 1991), Sist. *pal* 'ear (of corn); branch of a tree' (AFŠĀR SISTĀNI 1986), *plung* 'small heap [*xarman-e kučak va mohaqqar*] (of barley, corn or even fodder), either threshed or not threshed', Gil. *pil* 'thorns of rice or corn ear' (PĀYANDE 1987: 635), etc. We could add here a few words for 'stick' or similar objects, such as Prs. *pel*, Nāi. *pel* 'the piece of wood which is struck in the game of tip-cat (in Prs. *alak dulak*)', IrĀz.-Tāl. *pel* 'wooden crowbar' (ABDOLI 2001), Kerm. *pal* 'shepherd stick', etc. All or some of them might belong to the lexical family under discussion.

As far as the anatomical lexicon is concerned, worth noting is a word for 'finger' found in Fārs, which could be related to Krd. *pil/pîlk*. This is Dav. *peling* (SALĀMI 2002), *piling* (SALĀMI 2004: 64), Šir. *peleng*, Kāz. *piling* 'finger'. In his list of IrĀz. words occurring in written texts, ADIB TUSI (1992) quotes *pal* 'arm' (no. 1904) cross-referring to *pel* 'small stick used to play *alak dulak*' (no. 1554). In the Māz. variety spoken in Āmol, *pele* is 'arm [*bayal*]'.

Šir. *peleng* also occurs in the idioms *peleng zadan* 'to finger' and *sar-e peleng budan* 'to be happy' (see also Zarq. *sar-e peleng* (*bidan*) '(to be) happy'). In Širāzi, one also finds *pel* in *pel* (also *pelpel*) *zadan* 'to struggle [*dast-o-pā zadan*]' (XAZDUZ 2002: 72–73) and in the copulative compound *dast-o-pel* 'hand/arm'. In his repertoire of Colloquial Persian, MONTEIL (1954) mentions *pal* 'main; doigt' as an argot form (*lāti*) found in the expression *dast-o-pal* 'les mains' (from Sādeq Hedāyat); however, he considers this argot expression as a variant of Coll.Prs. *dast-o-bāl* 'arms and legs (of human beings)'. In NAJAFI 1999, *dast-o-pal*, equivalent in meaning to *dast-o-par*, is given as 'arms (of human beings)', and by extension, 'arms and legs; arms and face'; see also Dašt. *des-e pel* 'hands and face' (*des-e pelete bušur* "wash your hands and your face"), Buš. *dast-o-pal* 'struggle [*dast-o-pā*]', Xuns. *das-peleng* 'medium, means' (AŠRAF ALKETĀBI 1983: 442), which can be connected with Krmnš. *das-o-pel(eng)* etc. cited above. Further compounds, probably also containing *pel*-forms, are Badaxš. *pišpila* 'palm of the hand' (ŠĀLČI 1991), Bxt. (ČLang) *palmačča* 'hand, fingers and palm of the hand', Bxt. *par peleng* 'finger tip', Prs. *pal-o-pā* 'foot', Lo. *pelepiz* 'calf of the leg; leg (thigh and shank) [*par-o-pāče*]'. I would not exclude the possibility of reconsidering Prs. *pel* 'heel', which HENNING (1939: 98), «on account of its *l* from *d*», explained as an Eastern (Sogdian) lw. in New Persian, having replaced a «genuine Prs. *pai*», and reinterpret it as a form of our *pal-/pil-*family.

It is quite easy to understand how words for 'snap of the fingers' or 'fillip' can derive from words originally meaning 'finger' or 'part of a finger'. From SouthKrd. *pîlk* derives *pîlke* 'fillip'. Similarly, one finds Šir. *pelengak,* Zarq. *peleng(ak)*, Sarv. *peleng*, Buš. *peleng(ak)* (and its metathesized variant *pengalak*), Lārest. (Lār., Ger.) *pelenga*, Fin. *pelenga*, Bast. *pelenǰo āškāstâi* 'fillip; snap of finger'. See also Prs. *pelengak* 'sound of fingers'. Should one add here Farām. *pelek* 'to lick one's own fingers [*angošt lisidan*]'?

To conclude, I will mention Bal. *palk* 'forearm', which I recorded from a Bal. speaker native to Noške. Since Bal. *palk* 'forearm' has not been confirmed by any other Bal. speakers, and available dictionaries and glossaries do not record it, one could suspect that its presence in my informant's idiolect was due to an interference with Brahui, his mother-tongue (in fact, he is bilingual). While Bal. *palk* is recorded as 'sheet of metal or wood (used as door shutter); keel', Br. *palk* means (1) 'plank' and (2) 'pipe-bone of the forearm'. ROSSI (1979: A276) inserts Br. *palk* in his list A, containing Br. borrowings from Balochi. But if the sense 'plank' is common to both Br. *palk* and Bal. *palk* ('sheet of wood or metal'; see ELFENBEIN 1990-II, BARKER – MENGAL 1969, SAYAD HASHMI 2000), how would Brahui have developed the meaning 'pipe-bone of the forearm', not attested in Balochi? [74] Marw Bal. *palk* also means 'piece' and the iterative expression *palk palk* is used to say 'in pieces, in splinters' (ELFENBEIN 1963; see e.g. Marw Bal. *dār palk palk int* 'the wood is in pieces'); cf. SouthKrd. *pal* 'piece' (SAFIZĀDE 2001) above and perhaps (with a different formative) Bard. *pilāšk pilāšk* 'to bits (mainly said of dried wood to be burnt)'. A semantic development 'plank' → 'piece' (or *vice versa*) is however not obvious, nor is easy to link 'plank' and '(pipe-bone of the) forearm'. In any case, if Br. *palk* 'pipe-bone of the forearm' is Iranian,[75] as I assume, one should perhaps search outside Balochi to find its source. This matter, however, is beyond the scope of the present work.

3.6. At first sight, Yγn. *pax* 'finger' appears isolated in Iranian. Besides *pax*, we find its side-form (a derivative?) *páxa* 'the five fingers/the palm'

---

[74] See also Skt. *phálaka-* 'board', on whose etymology there is no agreement; cf. CDIAL 9053, EWA II: 202 (where the attribution to PHAL 'to burst' remains as dubious as it was in KEWA II). TURNER and MAYRHOFER do not refer to any Ir. forms.

[75] After the inclusion of Br. *palk* in a Dr. group ← IA proposed in DBIA 257, which justifies its exclusion from DED^2, this word has been not commented any more.

(ANDREEV – PEŠČEREVA 1957), 'the four fingers, thumb excluded' (XROMOV 1972), *paxxa* 'the five fingers' (MIRZOZODA 2008). The semantic relationship between *pax* and *páxa* is unclear to me; I cannot understand why *paxa* would convey in itself the notion of plurality, referring to all the fingers of a hand, as the Russian and English definitions provided by ANDREEV – PEŠČEREVA, XROMOV and MIRZOZODA let think. On the other side, the entry *paxxa* 'finger' in MIRZOZODA – QOSIMI 1995, the Taj. equivalents (namely, *angušt, lelak, panǰa*) and the Yγn. examples provided by MIRZOZODA 2008 (see for instance *awi uxš paxxayi ast* 'he has six fingers', s.v. *paxxa*), the Yγn. names of individual fingers containing *páxa*, for which see below, all run counter this assumption.

At my knowledge, no proposal has been advanced so far to etymologize Yγn. *pax*(*a*). In what follows I will try to suggest, even if with many reservations, possible connections with other Ir. words on the basis of predictable conceptualization patterns.

In Av. *Vd.* (9.14) one finds the adjectival compound *nava-pixa-* 'mit neuen Knoten' (BARTHOLOMAE 1904), describing a peculiar feature of a stick used in ritual functions. In correspondence with it, the Phl. translation has '9 *pixag*'. Since *9 pixag* is glossed with '9 *grēh*', one might deduce that *pixag* was not recognized as a current term at the time of the translation and/or commentary: it required therefore further explanation. It could be, e.g., an Av. word in Phl. garb (and in this case the existence in Middle Persian of a word sounding *pixag* and meaning 'knot' would be excluded), or it could be an areally (or otherwise) connoted word. In fact, a graphic sequence which may be read *pixag* occurs several times in different Phl. texts, always in the phrase *pad pixag šustan*, and always in connection with ceremonies of purification. But the reading and therefore the interpretation of this sequence remains disputable and no general agreement has been reached so far.

The reading *pyxk* ('[the stick of nine] knots') advanced by TAVADIA in the *Šāyest nē-šāyest* for a word «always written p aak, as if *pēšak*» (1930: 9–10 [13]) has been challenged by HENNING (1937: 92), who suggests reading *pyšk* and translating 'membrum', with reference to Sgd. *pyšyy* 'id.'[76] For the

---

[76] In Man. Sgd. one finds the graphic variants *pyšyy* and *pyš'k*; see also Buddh. Sgd. *'stkpyš'y* '(bony) limb'. Here belong SouthKrd. *pêše*, Awr. *peša* [= Sinnai], Biz. *pīšä* (MAZRAᶜTI *et al.* 1995), Dav. *pešek* 'bone' and Bast. *pešāk,* Farām. *pešak* 'wrist'. Though with many reservations, one is tempted to connect here also Sgd. *pyšnw* (reading not compelling), occurring in the list of body limbs edited in SUNDERMANN 2002: 143, for which SUNDERMANN, just as a guess, suggests translating 'forearm', «as beside '(upper) arm' and 'elbow' a word for 'forearm' may be expected» (ibid., fn. 63). In that list the word for

subsequent interpretations of the relevant passages, HENNING's siding has been crucial but not decisive, having been accepted by some scholars and rejected by others. Criticism is in TĀVUSI 1986: 143, while MAZDĀPUR (1990: 52 n. 53) lists the reasons which should lead to prefer the reading *pēšag* 'membrum'. According to KAPADIA (1953: 464), our Phl. word, which he reads *pîšak*, «originally means a Knot in a stick and it implies, as a part of the whole, the particular religious ceremonial of washing or purification, after pollution, more especially after contact with a dead body. The chief implement in this purificatory ablution is a *pîšak*, a stick of nine knots, to which a ladle of lead or iron is attached to pour out *gomêz* (sanctified urine of a bull) on the contaminated person. The idiom [...] (pa-pîšak-šôstan) refers to this *Barasnum* ceremony». A detailed description of the same instrument is given by KOTWAL (1969) in his *Supplementary texts to the Šāyest nē-šāyest*: «a nine knotted stick, technically called *naw-girē*; among the Parsis a kostīg is tied with nine knots round a bamboo stick to which a leaden spoon is attached. Nīrang, āb and xāk (fine gravel) are poured during the *barašnūm* ceremony». There, the name of the instrument is given as *pixag*, and not *pē/īšag* (see *Glossary*, s.v. *pixag*). KOTWAL's transliteration of the word (*pyyhk*; XII.27[77]) rests on the fact that the signs HENNING reads *š* may be read *yh* as well; according to GIGNOUX (1984: 184 n. 1), *pyyhk*, which he proposes as a different reading of the sequence previously read *pyšk* ('occupation, business') in the *Ardā Wīrāz Nāmag*, ch. 38, is «une graphie défective mais usuelle pour *pyhk*, *pyxg* 'noeud', abréviation pour *nō-pixag* (= av. *nava-pixəm*) : '(bâton) à neuf noeuds' utilisé dans la cérémonie

---

'wrist' is also lacking; but how to explain the final *-nw* ? In the same dialectal area of Bast. and Farām. (SE Iran), *pešak* appears to have developed the meaning of 'muscle'; cf. Lārest. (Lār., Ger.) *pešak-pâ* 'calf of the leg' and *pešake-das* 'biceps' [unless the latter lexicaled phrase should not be analyzed as containing the word for 'cat']. As for the actual status of MPrs. *pēšag* 'limb', note the asterisk marking as doubtful the headword **pēšag* 'limb, member, part' in MACKENZIE 1971; cf. also KAPADIA 1953: 464. Whatever may be the state of affairs in Pahlavi, which is (if any) the relationship between the lexical group for 'limb' of Sgd. *pišē,* Krd. *pêše*, etc. and Av. *pištra-*, MPrs. *pēšag*, Prs. *piše* 'profession, caste', etc. ? The close analogy between the human body and the social body, both made up by different parts, is repeatedly stressed in the Phl. literature (see for example GIGNOUX – TAFAZZOLI 1993: 169, 18). May we recognize here a metaphorical extension from a source SOCIETY to a target BODY? Or should we envisage a connection between the anatomical *piše*-group and Zarq. *piše* 'hollow cane', for which see below, p. 73?

77 The quoted passage proves that our Phl. word denotes an instrument, and not a generic body limb which has to be purified; the usage of the *pixag* avoids the contamination of the bowl containing *āb* and *gōmēz*.

du *baršnūm*. Le mot désigne par extension la cérémonie elle-même». GIGNOUX' stance on this matter is also adopted by VAHMAN (1986: 254; see there for further literature). It could be added however that a few modern "dialectal" words for 'reed' might support HENNING's reading <pyšk> (but not his translation); e.g. Zarq. *piše* 'hollow cane, also used as a device in medical practice'.

To Av. *pixa-*[78] and Phl. *pixag* belong Khwar. *pyxk* 'node' (HENNING 1956: 436)[79] and, in the body lexical domain, Man. Prth. *pw(x)g* 'joint (of the body)' (HENNING 1937: 87), occurring twice in the Manichaean hymn *Angad Rōšnān* in syntagmatic connection with the word for 'digit': *angušt puxag* (l. 11a) "joints of [my] toes" and *harwēn puxag čē dast ud angušt* (l. 12a) "each joint of [my] hands and of [my] fingers" (BOYCE 1954: 122-123). The Sgd. translation accompanying the Prth. text of this last verse reads *'rṯmy s'ṯ δsṯy 'ṯy 'ngwšṯy pyxt* (ibid., fn. 4).[80] As already dubitatively suggested by BENVENISTE (1940: 229: «*pyγ* peut-être av. *pixa* « nœud »»), the same Sgd. word could also be found in P14, l. 26. Unfortunately, the text is badly damaged; it is certain, however, that the topic of the relevant passage is about fingers and their movements. I would add here even Prs. *pekk* 'joint of fingers or toes',[81] as well as Rod. *pik* 'to stretch one's own finger towards someone else as a gesture of mockery'.

The pl. ending *-t* of Man. Sgd. *pyxt* in the line quoted above points to a heavy stem; *-y-* should represent a long vowel.[82] Connecting Sgl. *pēx*, Ydγ. *pīx* 'span from thumb to index-finger' (< **paixa-*) to Av. *pixa-* 'knot, joint in a reed', MORGENSTIERNE (IIFL-II: 242) postulated two different protoforms with vocalic alternation. Should we reconsider Phl. *pyyhk*, interpreting it not as «une graphie défective» (GIGNOUX), but as a variant of *pyhk/pyxk* with a long vowel?

---

78 To this Av. word TREMBLAY (2005: 180) doubtfully refers Pšt. *pəx* 'scab' ("Etym. unknown" in EVP; absent in NEVP).

79 See also *byxk, byxyk* "Knoten (im Schilfrohr; Zwinge (?, an der Lanze)" in BENZING – TARAF 1983, where a reference to Prs. *bēx* 'id.' is also made (but Prs. *bix* [*bēx*] means "root, bottom" and should be kept apart).

80 According to SIMS-WILLIAMS (1983: 44), *pwx-ty*, quoted in HENNING 1937: 87, «appears to be a superseded reading of this same form».

81 EILERS (1979-II: 717) suggests a connection between Prs. *pekk* and the form *päkk* occurring in the Gz. syntagmatic compound *päkk-o-pölü* 'Rippen und Kreuz', also found in Prs. (*pakk-o-pahlu*) and in several dialects («Dabei ist *päkk* eventuell identisch mit np. *pik* 'Gelenk'»). I would rather consider Gz. *päkk-o-pölü* as the result of a special and very productive Ir. lexical device which produces alliterative compounds of the type C*ak*-(*o*-)C.. (where C represents any initial consonant); see FILIPPONE 2006: 370.

82 Cf. Sgd. *pīx* in GHARIB 1995.

The mental association between JOINT OF THE BODY and JOINT OF A PLANT (with 'joint' I mean not only the place where two parts [bones or vegetal segments] meet, but also the part or space included between two articulations, knots or nodes) does not require much explanation, being a cognitive salient and privileged conceptualization path; several instances may be quoted of single Ir. words denoting (at a synchronic or a diachronic level) both the knuckles (or the phalanxes) of fingers and the knots in a stalk; I will mention in what follows just some of them.

Cognates of MPrs. *grēh*, quoted above as a gloss to the alleged MPrs. *pixag*, are Prs. *gereh* 'knot, as in a thread or on wood, etc.; knuckle; articulation', Kāz. *gere*, Yzd-JPrs. *gere* 'joint', Dašt. *gerend-e pinǰe*, Dežg. *gerend-e penǰa*, Zarq. *geren e angošt* 'finger joint', Krd. *girê* 'knot; knot/joint of a reed; joint of a finger' (South.Krd. HAŽĀR 1990, Kurm. KURDOEV 1960; see also CABOLOV 2001 with etymological notes), KurmKrd. also *geh* 'finger joint', etc. Derivatives from the same root, also belonging to the anatomical lexicon, are MPrs. *gračag*, Man. Prth. *grehčag* (SUNDERMANN 2003: 220), Krd. *girêčik* (South.Krd. HAŽĀR 1990, Kurm. RIZGAR 1993), ZorYzd. *grænǰ, græng* (MAZDĀPUR 1995 s.v. *band*) 'joint, knuckle'.

Bal. *bog* (EBal. *boγ*) 'joint; finger knuckle; vertebra' (MAYER 1910; ELFENBEIN 1990-II, etc.)[83] belongs to both the botanic and the anatomical domain; the same senses have been recorded for Jir.-Kahn. *bûg, bûγ*. The Bal. compound *gulbog* (with *gul* 'flower'), occurring in a SBal. version of the epic ballad on the death of Dodā of the Gorgeǰ tribe, labelled in BARKER – MENGAL's *Glossary* as 'literary in Raxšāni' (1969 II: 290, l. 39), is a poetical term for 'finger'. A further instance of the metaphorical connection KNOT IN STALK = JOINT is provided by MORGENSTIERNE (IIFL-II: 242), who, in order to justify the proposed connection between Sgl. *pēx*, Ydγ. *pīx* and Av. *pixa-*, quotes Skt. (RV) *párvan-* 'knot; joint' and its outcomes in modern IA (see also CDIAL 7947; EWA II: 99f.).

There is a group of words denoting the stubble, i.e. the pointed, dry stalks of corn and barley remaining on the ground after the harvest, which could be associated to Av. *pixa-* and cognates. These are: Xor. (Kelidar) *pīx* (ŠĀLČI 1991), (TrbHayd.) *pux, puxal*, (Her.) *puxa* 'chaff', (dial.) Taj. *paxol* (Kara-Tegin) 'straw', (Badaxš.) 'rush, reed' (ROZENFEL'D 1982), Haz. *pʌxʌl* 'straw', Sist. *paxāl*,[84] Birǰ. *paxal*, 'reaped corn and barley', Qāi. *pɛxɛl* 'stalks of corn and barley', Yγn. (also dial. Taj.) *pĭx, pĭnx* 'splinter', *pīx* 'thorn, a thorny plant' (MIRZOZODA 2008). At first sight, it seems that this lexical

[83] Cf. also Br. *bog* 'joint in sugarcane, cereals, etc.'.

[84] See also Sist. *paxali* 'stubble-field' (RAXŠĀNI 1981: 113).

cluster has a prevalent diffusion in Eastern Persian, though traces of it are also found in the Central Plateau dialect area and in Southern Iran;[85] cf. Zar. *pəxal*, Sirǰ. *pexal* 'what remains of the stalks of corn after harvesting', Kerm. *pexal* 'scraps of paper and straw; rubbish on the water', Jir.-Kahn. *paxal* 'rubbish'.[86] To this group, another may be associated, denoting pointed protuberances in animal bodies, such as AfγPrs. *pīx*, Išk. *pex* 'spur of bird', Birǰ. *paxol* 'paw of cat or dog'. Sist. *pix* is said of human teeth, when they are reminiscent of a dog's teeth, or when they are ground with angry, while *pixol* means 'nail, in particular the nail of animals like cats'. In the West of the Ir. plateau, one finds Tehr. *pax zadan* (*kardan*) 'to scratch (of a piece of wood, iron or similar thing)' (ADIB TUSI 1963–1964) and Dašt. *čang-o pexel* 'fighting with claw; scratching someone's face and head'.

All this considered, I think that assuming Yγn. *pax* 'finger' as the result of a metaphoric process (with SEGMENT OF A VEGETABLE as the source and SEGMENT OF A FINGER as the target), and a subsequent metonymic extension (→ FINGER), is a guess we could hazard.

3.7. Ar. *qaṣab,* whose primary meaning is 'cane, reed', if used with reference to the human body, denotes all hollow channels or tubular bones, like windpipe, trachea, or shinbone; speaking of a finger (*qaṣab-ul-iṣbaᶜ*), it refers to its phalanxes. Similarly, Prs. *qasab*, a well integrated Ar. loanword, is used to refer to different parts of the human body, in particular the hollow ones, like bones and veins ('windpipe; the bones of the fingers; finger; lachrymal ducts' STEINGASS 1963).[87] The sense of 'finger', given by STEINGASS beside that of 'bones of the finger', is probably due to a misunderstanding or to an occasional metonymic extension.

4.1. Engl. *finger* and its Germanic cognates are prevalently explained as derived from the notion FIVE (IE **penkʷe* 'five' > **penkʷ-ro-* 'finger'). The 'five'-etymology (first advanced by F. BOPP) still remains the most ac-

---

[85] If (Fārs) Dav. *pifâl* 'straw, sweeping' does belong here, it should be added to the rather long list of words with *x* > *f* in Iranian. That *x*, *xw* > *f* is a natural phonetic change, largely found outside Iranian as well, has already been stated (see e.g. EILERS 1988: 59 f.) but the subject is still to be treated in its complexity.

[86] See also Kerm. *pexeli*, Zar. *pəxəli*, etc. 'stubble-field'. Possibly, the notion CHOPPED STRAW is associated to RUBBISH and successively, to DIRT, as proved by Kerm. *pexal o pexâl* 'bird droppings', Abiā. *paqal* 'donkey manure', etc.

[87] See also *qasabe* 'reed; bone', *qasabe-ye kobrā* 'tibia', *qasabatorrie* 'windpipe', *qasabe-ye soqrā* 'fibula', the last two labelled as "ancien" by LAZARD 1990a.

cepted, though alternative etymologies have been advanced. The 'five'-etymology supporters are listed in HOPTAM 2000: 77 (and n. 1), 86–87, together with the other etymologies put forward to that date.[88]

In any case, relationship or even identity between words for 'five' and those for 'hand' have been observed in several languages.[89] For this association both directions are possible.

MPrs. *panǰag* is an *-*aka*-derivative from *panǰ* 'five'; it denotes the human hand/foot (and by extension the animal paw/claw), pointing to the five fingers as a whole. The same senses are conveyed by Prs. *panǰe*, which may denote the whole hand (*panǰe-ye dast*, including the palm, from the wrist to the fingertips), the foot (*panǰe-ye pā*), or the five fingers (or toes), perceived as expanded or tightly curled up into a clenched fist.[90] Prs. *xamse* 'five; the five fingers, the hand' is an Ar. loanword (cf. Ar. *xamsa* 'five'), sharing the same conceptual motivation.

Cognates of Prs. *panǰe* are widespread in Iranian; however, all these forms (Par. *peñǰa, penǰa, panǰa* 'the five fingers of the hand; paw', *peñǰa-e påika* 'the five fingers of the foot', Wx. *panǰá* 'wrist; the five fingers of the hand', Pšt. *panǰá* 'the hand; the five fingers, the palm; the foot; claw, paw', Yγn. *pánǰa* 'the five fingers' (also 'middle finger'), Šγn. *panǰā* 'the five fingers of the hand and the five toes of the foot', Yzγ. *panǰa* 'palm of the hand with open fingers') etc. are loanwords from Persian/Tajik. Of course, *panǰe*-forms may display areal phonetic peculiarities, such as voicing of initial *p* in some Central dialects (cf. Esf-JPrs. *banǰe*, Varz. *banǰe* ['patte du chat'], etc., in accordance with the voicing of initial *p* in words for 'five' and derivatives (cf. Ard. *bāń* '5', *bāǰe* '50', Tār. *banǰ* '5', *banǰā* '50', etc.), or loss of internal nasal, like SouthKrd. *pêǰî*, Lārest. *peǰ* (for which see below). Single forms may present semantic peculiarities, as Del. *payn̦ǰae*, which means 'the five fingers', but also 'glove' and 'everything in number of five'.

Besides the many *-*aka*-derivatives of words for 'five', such as MPrs. *panǰag*, Prs. *panǰe*, Bal. *panǰa(g)*,[91] etc., there are also -*ā*/*o*/*ul*-formations

[88] Among these, there is HOPTAM's personal etymology, with Engl. *finger* and cognates tentatively (and to my opinion, not convincingly enough) explained as belonging to a sound-symbolic lexical group (*f*- or *fl*-words, denoting a to and fro movement).

[89] See also above, p. 43.

[90] No mention will be done here of the several semantic extensions grounded on metaphorical associations in domains other than the body domain.

[91] In ELFENBEIN 1983a: 146, read *panǰa* instead of *panǰaw* (-*w* is a labial glide preceding the obl. marker -*ā* in *panǰawā*). The meaning 'hand' is preferable to 'fist' (proposed by

that in most cases designate an animal body part ('claw, paw') and imply an ironic or derogatory attitude if referred to human beings. These are: (colloquial) Prs. *panǰul* 'paw of cat or the like' (FF, NAJAFI 1999),[92] Esf.Prs. *pangāl*, Šir. *penǰāl*, Zarq. *pangāl, penǰāl*, Xor. *pengāl*,[93] Birǰ. *pangol, pangul*, TrbHayd. *pangal*, Her. *panǰōl*, Šušt. *pangul,* Lo. *pangāl*, Nāi. *penǰul* ('the fingers of the hand, often used in a derogatory sense'), Del. *paynǰūlae* (also 'the five fingers'), Qm. *panǰule*, Kerm. *pangol* ('paw; human nails when they are long (used as a joke or an insult)'), Abiā. *panǰula*, Yzd. *pængol*, Xur. *panǰul*, Rāv. *panγol*, Bard. *pangor, pangur*, Sirǰ. *pangor*, Damāv. *panqāl*, Šahr. *pangâl*, Māz. (Sār.) *panǰul*, *pangōl*, KurmKrd. *pencero<u>k</u>* (and by metathesis *perinco<u>k</u>* RIZGAR 1993), etc.

The usage of these *l*-derivatives in connection with the human body does not always (or everywhere) imply a negative attitude of the speaker towards his/her addressee. AfγPrs. *panǰāl* and Biz. *panǰule* (MAZRA^{c}TI *et al.* 1995), for instance, has the same semantic implications as Prs. *panǰe*, which is both 'human hand' and 'paw'. According to SAFIZĀDE 2001, SouthKrd. *panǰu<u>l</u>a* means 'the hand with the five fingers, from the wrist to the fingertips',[94] while Bxt. *pangal* refers to 'the five fingers stuck together and kept outstretched, prepared to receive something'; see also ČLang *panga, pangâl* 'paw; hand; the five fingers'.

SCHWARTZ (1992: 424ff.) has explained Prs. *pang* 'cluster of dates' as «the regular outcome of PIE *$ponk^{w}o$-», with the meaning 'pertaining to the hand' (the proposal would reconcile Prs. *pang* with Pol. *pęk* and Russ. *puk* 'bundle, etc.'). In fact, given the close link between HAND and PART OF TREE, one might also directly assume, at least for Iranian, a lexical innovation based on a semantic change ('hand' → 'bundle, etc.', with subsequent phonetic differentiations).[95] To Prs. *pang* 'bundle', one may add the follow-

---

ELFENBEIN in the *Glossary*; see e.g. ibid.: 102–103 (l. 66) *do sad muhr kutag-iš panǰawā wāz* «two hundred mohrs he put in his open hand»).

92 Other Prs. dictionaries only record the sense of 'scratch, scraping'.

93 MONCHI-ZADEH (1990: no. 422) explains the internal *-g-* (instead of *-ǰ-*) in this group of words as resulting from a contamination with *pang* 'Stock, Rute'. Why not an analogical change based on *čang(āl)*?

94 HAŽĀR 1990 cites this word with the meaning of 'delicate and small hand'.

95 Cognates of Prs. *pang* in the same botanic sense are largely recorded in Iranian. As far as we are concerned here, the question of the original meaning of *$penk^{w}$- is negligible (both '5' → 'hand' → subsequent extensions, and 'hand' → subsequent extensions [including 'hand' → '5'] are pathways fitting well our reasoning), though the hypothesis of an original meaning 'hand' remains attractive, indeed.

ing: Bxt. *peng, pang,*[96] Lārest. (Gerāši) *peǰ*, Ār.-Bidg. *pə:ǰ*, having the same meaning as Prs. *panǰe* ('the hand, the five fingers'). Farām. *penǰ* and Bal. *panč* are recorded with the meaning of 'fist';[97] Sarv. *penǰ,* Mās. *penǰ* (SALĀMI 2004: 153) and Zarq. *penǰ* belong to the dimensional domain and refer to the quantity which a hand may grasp ('handful'). One could also add Lārest. *pengi* 'small quantity of anything' (ADIB TUSI 1963–1964).

Šir. *penǰ* is given as 'fingers of the hand' in XADIŠ 2000 (as opposed to *penǰe* 'fingers and toes', but this differentiation seems to be contingent on the lexicographer's interpretation) and as 'claw, talon' in BEHRUZI 1969; 'claw, talon' is also the meaning of Zā. *penc* (TODD 1985),[98] Šušt. *pang*, Buš. *penǰ,* Lir.-Dayl. *penǰ* (LIRĀVI 2001: 251). A metonymical association is responsible for the sense acquired by Sist. *peng*, which is a denomination for 'the high part of the back' (from which *pengi* 'a load born on the shoulder' derives).

In the dialects spoken in Hormoz, Rodān and Fin, *penǰ* is 'nail'; the same meaning is conveyed by SBšk. (Garu) *penč*, NBšk. (Senderk, Angohrān) *penč*[99] and Bal. *pinč*, which I recorded from Bal. speakers native to southern Ir. Balochistan and from a Baloch living in Oman (native to Pakistani Makrān). In particular, according to a Bal. speaker from Kasrākand, *pinč* denotes that part of the fingernail which grows disjunct from the flesh, *i.e.*, the part which has to be periodically cut. This latter sense reminds the 'long nail' of Kerm. *pangol*. Bal. *pinč* 'nail' is also recorded in AYYUBI 2002 (*penč*, labelled Makrāni), SAYAD HASHMI 2000 and ZAND MOQADDAM 1991: 380. This set of words for 'nail' also include KurmKrd. *pencik* 'Fingernagel' (OMAR 1992).

From SAYAD HASHMI 2000 we learn that Bal. *pinč* 'nail' is "erroneously" used "in many places" with the meaning of 'finger'. This information finds no confirmation in the data I have collected; however, there is no reason to question it. An alleged Bal. *pinč* 'finger' would find its collocation side by side with many cognate words used with (or *also* with) this sense and widespread in Central and Southern Kurdish, in some Lori areas, in Central dialects and in South Iran (Fārs and Lārestān), as well as in some Eastern varieties of Persian.

---

96 See also Bxt. *pang, panǰ* 'talons' in LORIMER 1922.

97 Cf. *panč* in SAYAD HASHMI 2000 ('the five fingers bent in order to punch someone') and (Sarāwāni and Lāšāri) *penč* 'wrist [Prs. *moč*]' in a handwritten draft (letters *alef – ǰim*) of an (Ir.)Bal. dictionary compiled by ABDUL HAMID and kindly put by the author at disposal of the *Balochi Comparative Etymological Dictionary Project* directed by A.V. ROSSI at the University of Naples L'Orientale – IsIAO Rome.

98 Cf. also Siverek *pänǰ* in HADANK 1932: 163.

99 From G. BARBERA's unpublished material. According to BARBERA (2004), even in Mināb the word for 'nail' is *penǰ*; see also above, fn. 61.

These are: SouthKrd. *panǰ* (SAFIZĀDE 2001), *panǰa* (also 'the five fingers with the palm of the hand; paw'), SorKrd. *pence,* SulKrd. *pence* (also 'hand, paw'),[100] Abd. *penǰe, penǰeri* (ŽUKOVSKIJ 1922: 110), Anār. *penǰa*, Frv. *penǰe*, Siv. *penǰe* (LECOQ 1979), Xur. *penǰå*, Ardest. *banǰi* (*bonǰī* in BAILEY 1933–1935: 773), Tār. *banǰa*, Keš. *banǰa*, Šušt. *panǰe* (also 'the five fingers'), BoirAhm. *penǰa*,[101] Mamas., Dāreng., Dorun., Kal. (Lor), Nud., Somγ., Ban., Pāp., Dusir., Rič., Gorgn., Mosq., Kuz. *penǰa*, Kal. (Tāǰ.) *penǰar*, Kurdšuli *penǰe* (MORGENSTIERNE 1960: 133),[102] Gavk. *penǰa*, Dav. *pinǰa*, Zarq. *penǰe* ('finger or toe'), Mās., Kuz., Dahl., Knd., Baliā. *penǰa,* Kāz. *penǰe*,[103] Dežg., Birov., Hay., Dādenǰ. *penǰe*, Buš. *penǰe*, Lir.-Dayl. *pinǰe*, Dašt. *pinǰe* and proceeding eastwards, Xonǰi *penǰa,* Lār. *penǰa* (KAMIOKA – RAHBAR – HAMIDI 1986). In Koroši, the Bal. dialect spoken in Fārs, one also finds *penǰa* 'finger'.

While in literary Tajik *panǰa* denotes the hand (or the foot) as a whole (i.e. the five fingers and the palm, or the five toes and the sole), in Southern Tajik *panǰa* also means 'finger' (ROZENFEL'D 1982; Badaxš. *panǰa* 'the open hand; finger, first finger'); see also Kāb. *painǰa* 'les 5 doigts, doigt' (FARHÂDI 1955: 102) and Sist. *penǰol* 'finger'. Loanwords (from some Eastern Persian variety) are Par. *panǰâ* (IIFL-I), Yγn. *pánǰa*, which, besides 'the five fingers', also means 'middle finger',[104] as well as *pänǰäla* 'finger' recorded in a Turkish dialect spoken in North-Eastern Xorāsān (Langar) (DOERFER – HESCHE 1993: 171).

Once the consciousness of the original link between the notion FIVE and words meaning 'finger' (passing through HAND) went lost, new denominations for 'hand' were created, as is shown by (dial.) Taj. *panǰ-panǰa* 'palm' (← 'the five fingers') (ROZENFEL'D 1982) or Buš. *panǰ penǰe* 'the five fingers'. These two expressions are lexical innovations corresponding in meaning to Prs. *panǰe*. However, *panǰ penǰe* may be used with the meaning 'the five fingers' even in Persian, as attested by the following expression occurring in ŠĀMLU 2000: 1011: *panǰ penǰe-at rā ^{c}asal koni dahān (-e folāni) begozāri, angošthā-yat rā az bix mikonad* "should you dip your five fingers

[100] The *panǰe*-type 'finger' seems to be a lexical feature of the Central/South. Krd. area; see however *pence* 'Finger' in OMAR 1992 (Kurmancî).

[101] According to ANONBY (2003: 186), 'finger' in BoirAhm. is *k^{j}ilits*.

[102] Kurdšuli is the name of a small tribe speaking a Lori dialect, to which MORGENSTIERNE (1960: 133–134) devoted a few notes.

[103] 'Forefinger' according to BEHRUZI 2002; cf. below, p. 131.

[104] See below p. 140.

in the honey and put them into so-and-so's mouth, he would pull them up by the roots" (said in order to underline so-and-so's ungratefulness).[105]

4.2. The semantic range of Prs. *panǰe* and cognates, discussed in the preceding paragraph, presents many analogies with that of Prs. *čang* and derivatives/cognates, though the original notion on which the latter lexical cluster relies is seemingly quite different.

Prs. *čang* denotes anything hooked or bent (like hooks or similar objects); in the anatomical domain, it is 'claw of wild beast, talon of bird' and, in human beings, 'fingers somewhat crooked' or 'expanded hand'. The usage of *čang* for 'hand' is peculiar to the informal register (so LAZARD 1990a) and/or evocative of the idea of violence and rudeness (NAJAFI 1999); the instances collected in DEHX show that *čang* was already current in this sense in classical Persian poetry. Among *čang*-derivatives, *čangāl* is nowadays mostly used as the name of the pronged tool with which one eats food, i.e., the fork, or any other instruments with a similar form. It also denotes body parts like paws, talons, claws; therefore, *čangāl* (and similarly *čange, čangol, čangale*, etc.) is used with a specific reference to animals, in particular birds of pray, even if there is no shortage of examples in classical poetry (see some of them in DEHX) implying reference to human beings. This also happens with AfγPrs *čangāl*. According to NAJAFI 1999, when using Prs. *čangul* as 'hand, fist', the speaker wants to display his/her negative attitude (even contempt) towards the referent. In Tajik, one finds *čang* 'hand with crooked fingers', *čangol* 'hand', while *čangal, čangul* is reserved to predatory animals and birds of prey.

Prs. *čang* (with its derivatives), generally derived from IE **keng-*, **kenk-* 'hook' (IEW 537–538, mainly based on Germ. and Slav., apparently not IA), has several cognates in New Iranian, which belong to different semantic domains. Leaving out the senses of 'claw, talon' or 'paw', found virtually everywhere and attested in Ir. since ancient times (see Av. °*čingha-* in *Yt.* 5.113 *pæšō-čingha-* 'with spread claws'), I will focus in what follows on the human body lexicon only.

---

[105] BROWN (2005: 526–529) describes and comments (also including a useful map) the two ways in which languages may lexically treat the human finger and the hand: 1. identity (a single word denotes both 'hand' and 'finger' and/or 'fingers'; 2. differentiation (one word denotes 'hand' and another, different word denotes 'finger'). In consideration of *angošt* and *panǰe*, we may say that Persian represents a good example of both types.

A metaphorical mapping has produced words for '(human) nail' starting from *čang*-words for '(animal) nail': cf. (IrĀz.) Rudbār *čangâl* (LAZARD 1990b), Lo. *čangāl* (also 'hand'), Birǰ. *čangol*. The transfer from PAW to HAND and/or THE FIVE FINGERS OF THE HAND is quite common; beside Prs., cf. Birǰ. *čang* 'hand and fingers', *čangal, čangol* 'hand; claw', Gor. *čang, čangal* 'griffe (au sens figuré: main)' (MOKRI 1966), SouthKrd. *čing* 'the hand including all the fingers' (SAFIZĀDE 2001), Lo. *čangāl* (also 'nail'), Buš. *čang* 'the palm of the hand and the fingers', Fin. *čengāl* 'hand', *čangol* 'fist', Siv. *čäŋg* 'fist', Māz. (AliĀb.) *čangâl* 'hand, from the wrist to the fingertips', (Tabari) *čangāl* 'palm of the hand' (ADIB TUSI 1963–1964), etc. In EIr., *čang*-forms with an explicit reference to the hand or the totality of fingers are all (East.)Prs. loanwords; cf. Pšt. *čang, čangắl, čangúl* 'hand; the five fingers; claw, talon',[106] Yγn. *čank* 'paw; hand', *čangol* 'claw of birds of pray; hand', Wx. *čangol* 'paw; the five fingers of the hand; hand; arm', Šγn. *čāng* 'claw, paw; hand', etc.

The hollow of a hand, when its fingers are slightly bendy, works quite well as a container. There is a strong conceptual relation between a container and its content. Therefore several *čang*-forms are used as terms for weight measures. In DEHX, one finds *čang* and *čange* as synonyms of Prs. *mošt* and *daste* 'handful'. In Standard Persian of Iran, however, *čang* and *čange* 'handful' are not in use; *čang*-forms for 'handful' are found in the dialects of South Iran (Buš. *čang*, Dašt. *čang*, Lārest. (Xonji) *čang*, KAMIOKA – YAMADA 1979), in Eastern Persian (Sist. *čāng*, Her. *čang*), and in other Ir. languages as well; compare Krd. (Central, South.) *čing*, (Kurm.) *çeng*, Tāl. *čango, čangə*, Qasr. *čenga*, Gz. *čēŋg*, Nāi. *čeng* (*čeng-čenga* 'by handfuls'), Iran. Bal. (Makrān) *čangol* ('a handful of grass', AYYUBI 2002), Šγn. *čangol*, Baǰ. *čingol*, etc.[107] Elsewhere we find further semantic specializations, with *čang*-forms referring to the content of any matter which can be held in two hands, i.e. a 'double handful'. This is the case with Birǰ. *čangal* ('hand, claw', but also 'two cupped hands' and 'quantity contained in two cupped hands'), Qāi. *čɛngɛl*, Kerm. *čangâl*, Gil. *čange* ('the quantity of harvested

---

106 Pšt. *mangul* 'paw; talon' (also 'the five fingers, the hand including the five fingers' in RAVERTY 1860) is perhaps better explained as the (lexicalized ?) second element of an echo-compound (*čangul mangul*, with *m*-alternation), rather than as an outcome of **hamanguli-*, as proposed by MORGENSTIERNE in EVP, NEVP s.v. *grut*. This suggestion has already been advanced in DE CHIARA 2008 s.v. See also Xuns. *mäŋgūl*, which «erscheint zunächst nur als Reimwort zu *šängūl*», EILERS 1976 s.v.

107 See also Hi. *čungī* 'a cess levied from grain-sellers etc. (being as much as a man can grasp in his hand)' (PLATTS 1930). Ir. lw.?

rice contained in two hands'), Bal. *čank* (ELFENBEIN 1990-II, SAYAD HASHMI 2000),[108] Sariq. *čangul*, etc., all of the meaning 'double handful'.

In Pashto, Ossetic and Kurdish-Zāzā, *čang*-forms have developed the sense of 'arm' or 'part of arm'. Cf. Oss. *cong* 'arm',[109] KurmKrd. *çeng* 'arm (from the shoulder to the elbow); wing',[110] Zā. (Čabaxčur) *čäñgil* 'Achsel, Schulter' (HADANK 1932: 363), Pšt. *cangə́l, cəngə́l, cangə́lə, cəngə́lə, sangə́l* 'elbow; the arm from the elbow to the wrist' (see also *cāng* 'wing of a bird'), Ōrm. *caŋgʌl* 'elbow' (MORGENSTIERNE 1932b). Whether the sense of 'arm' derives from the conceptual association with HAND, or the element perceived as crooked is rather the elbow, is still to be defined.

Pšt. *cangə́l* shares the sense of 'elbow' with co-radical words in other Ir. languages.[111] On account of Phl. *ārešnčand* (*'lšnčnd*) (M 6) and *čandārešn* (*čnd 'lšn*) (K 20) 'as much as an ell (elbow)', which glosses Av. *čiąkazauatō* in *Farhang-ī Ōīm* iii, g. 5, HENNING (1945: 471 fn.3) corrected the reading of the odd Av. sequence and replaced it with *čiąkaδauatō*, considered as a bad spelling of **čąkaδavatō* 'of that which has an elbow, or forearm'. He reconstructs in this way an Av. form **čąkaδa*- 'ell, elbow', otherwise unattested, from which Pšt. *cangə́l* would derive.[112] A different emendation has

108 Br. *čank* 'double handful' is a lw. from Bal.

109 Oss. *cong* is also 'branch', according to a universal cognitive model equating the human body, which in this case represents the source domain, with that of a tree. See also Pšt. *cə́ngə, cāng* 'branch of a tree', Ōrm. *cāŋgə* 'branch'. Numberless examples could be added. I will limit myself to quoting Taj. *panǰa* 'branch'.

110 See also *hinçeng, hiçeng, piçeng* 'armpit'. For SouthKrd., HAŽĀR 1990 gives *čingiḻ* 'arm / armpit [*baɣal*]'.

111 I would challenge the connection of Xor. *zengeča, zīngīča* 'elbow' with Pšt. *cangə́l* suggested by MONCHI-ZADEH (1990: 206–207). Words for 'elbow' which may be considered as cognates to Xor. *zengeča* are found in Kermān dialects (Kerm. *zenče,* Bard. *zomče,* Rāv. *zamče,* Sirǰ. *zomče*) and in Tāleši (*dasi zīng,* PIREJKO 1976). In those linguistic areas, a *č*- > *z*- development may hardly be assumed, since the affricate *č* in initial position has a rather strong stability. Surely, any connection between Khot. *tcaṃgalai* (interpreted as *tcaṃgala* + *i* and translated 'his elbows' in BAILEY 1979) and Pšt. *cangə́l* is to be excluded. According to KUMAMOTO (1987a), on the basis of the text where *tcaṃgalai* occurs, the meaning 'elbow' is inadmissible; one should rather think to something like 'chains' instead.

112 See also NEVP 17; DE CHIARA 2008 (< **čangada*-; with further references). To Pšt. *cangə́l*, one should also connect Pšt. *cang* 'flank, side'.

been proposed by KLINGENSCHMITT (1968: 64): **ciṇkaδauuatō*, gen. sing. or acc. pl. of Av. **čiṇkaδa-* (< OIr. **čankada-* 'Armbeuge').[113]

Br. *čangulī* 'elbow' has been considered as an «assimilated LW < Pš (rather than < Prs *čangul*, °*gal* 'claw, hand')» (NEVP 17). This assumption could be right; one cannot rule out, however, that *čangulī* has been borrowed from an Ir. language other than Pashto, having a *čang*-word for 'elbow' not known in the literature (ROSSI 1979: F28).[114] Balochi should be excluded; there one finds *čāngoṭ* 'elbow' (SAYAD HASHMI 2000, RAZZAQ – BUKSH – FARRELL 2001); see also *čangot* 'elbow' in (Bal.) Koroši.

But let's come back to the core of our discussion, i.e. the Ir. terms for 'finger'. Among the several glosses listed in DEHX s.v. *čangāl*, one reads: 'anyone of the human fingers',[115] though no example illustrates this definition. To find a sure *čang*-type 'finger' we have to look to Sistāni, where we find *čongol*, the usual Sist. term for this part of the body.[116] Sistāni has influenced Balochi, in particular the Bal. varities spoken in Iran and in Marw (Turkmenistan); cf. Bal. *čangul*, *čangol* 'finger' in ELFENBEIN 1963, COLETTI 1981, FILIPPONE 2000–2003: 60–61; AYYUBI 2002 (Sarhaddi). To explain Bal. *čangul* 'finger', therefore, there is no reason to think to an Ur. loanword as suggested in KORN 2005: 293. Elsewhere in Balochi, *čangul* (also *čungal* RAZZAQ – BUKSH – FARRELL 2001) is used in the "usual" senses of 'claw of birds, paw of cats (or similar animals)' and 'fork'. To Sist. *čongol* and Bal. *čangul*, one may add the following: *čungl* 'finger' in the Tajik variety spoken by the Fārsivāns of Turkmenistan (MAHMUDOV 2001: 47), IrĀz. (Ker.) *čengil* 'finger' (ZOKĀ 1954), Gil. *čungul* 'the extremity of fingers or toes'. In Jiroft and Kahnuǰ, *čangol* means 'the distance between the fingers or the toes', entering therefore the measurement domain.

Xuns. *čongol* and Lo. *čangul* 'pinch' (RAHMĀNIĀN 2000: 83 fn. 1) also belong here.

---

113 I warmly thank R. SCHMITT for having brought to my notice KLINGENSCHMITT's position on the matter. In a personal communication, SCHMITT has also stressed the soundness of KLINGENSCHMITT's emendation (OIr. **cank*° > Av. **cink*°, not **cąk-*).

114 Note that *-ī*-derivatives in Ir. cognate words are also found elsewhere: cf. Aft. *čanguli*, Māz. (Sā.) *čangeli*, Ydγ. *čigāli* etc. 'claw, paw'.

115 See also 'finger' in STEINGASS 1963 s.v. *čangāl*.

116 In the *Qor'ān-e Qods*, the ms. containing a Qoran translation which for many aspects points to a Sistanic origin, <čngl> is only used with reference to animals: cf. (VI. 146) <hr xd'vnd čngly> (with *xudāvand* in the sense of 'having', common in Classic Persian) in correspondence to Ar. *kull ḏī-l-ẓufr*, ie. 'all (animals) having claws'. Cf. RAVĀQI 1985: 80 and fn. 5 (<čngl> 'undivided hoof [*som-e pā ke šekāfte nabāšad*]').

4.3. Among the Ir. words discussed at § 4.1, directly or indirectly correlated with the notion FIVE, there are a few words for 'nail'. For them, alternative associative paths may be assumed: FIVE → FIVE FINGERS → HAND → PAW, CLAW → NAIL, or FIVE → FIVE FINGERS / HAND → FINGER → NAIL.

The relationship between FINGER and NAIL is easily understandable on the basis of the nature and position of these body parts. The conceptual transfer may be bidirectional: words originally meaning 'finger' may acquire the meaning of 'nail' and *vice versa*, as it happened in the Central dialects, mainly in the Kermān area, where Kerm. *nāxun*, Rāv. *nāxūn*, Bard. *nāxun*, Zar. *nâxû*, Sirǰ. *nāxun*, Yzd. *nāxun*[117] are the current term for 'finger' (cf. Prs. *nāxon, nāxun* and cognates 'nail'). Here also belongs Sgl. *narxā̊k* 'nail', occurring in the lexicalized phrases *katta narxā̊k* 'thumb' (see below p. 103) and *pu-narxā̊k* 'toe' (IIFL-II, quoted with a question mark). Here should also belong Haz. *narxūn* 'forefinger' (if FOREFINGER ← FINGER ← NAIL; cf. below p. 131; a different explanation is given in DULLING 1973: «*xūn* probably stands for M. *xuruun* (= finger)»).

Bal. (Raxš.) *nāun*, (Keči) *nāxun*, *nākun* 'fingerbreadth' (← 'fingernail', ELFENBEIN 1992: 252) may be mentioned here. In a fieldwork conversation with a Bal. speaker from Nal (Xuzdār), I recorded *hor* (basically 'finger')[118] used several times for 'nail'. The same metonymical association is attested in the Turkish speaking area: in the Xorasanian Turk. dialect spoken at Xarw-e ᶜOlyā, for instance, *durnaq* is 'finger' (DOERFER – HESCHE 1993: 127); cf. Turk. *dirnaq* 'nail'. Similarly, in Zargari, a Romani dialect spoken in Zargar (near Qāzvin), *nāy* is both 'nail' and 'finger'.[119]

4.4. The metonymical association KNUCKLE → FINGER motivates a word for 'finger' documented in South and Central Kurdish: *qamk* 'finger, joint of finger' (*qâmiq* 'finger' SAFIZĀDE 2001), Mahâb. *qâmq*, Mukri *khamök* (CHRISTENSEN – BARR 1939: 306) 'finger', Sul. *qamk* 'thumb' (*qamk-y pê* 'big toe'),[120] Lo. *kāw-e pā* 'toe of the foot' (UNVALA 1958: 16).

These lexical forms belong to a very large WIr. family including words for different kinds of articulations (knucklebone, astragalus, wrist, elbow,

117 Information provided to me by H. REZĀI BĀFBIDI, whom I thank for his usual kindness.

118 See below, p. 90.

119 For this information I am indebted to H. REZĀI BĀFBIDI.

120 On 'finger' → 'thumb' see below p. 117. According to CHRISTENSEN – BARR (1939: 306), however, Sul. *k'amouk* is 'finger'.

ankle, heel, shinbone, knee, basin, etc.), as is the case with Prs. *qāb* 'knucklebone'.[121] As for the finger domain, in particular, the following terms are recorded as 'finger-joint': KurmKrd. *kab, k'ap* (*kaw* RIZGAR 1993), Lak. *qow kel̂ek,* Knd., Pāp., Dusir. *qâb*, Mās., Birov., Kuz. *qâv,* Mamas. *qâb-e k̂elič*, Abd. *qâb-e penǰe*, Rič., Somγ. *qâb-e penǰa*, Dav. *qâv-e pinǰe*, Mosq., Dādenǰ., Dāreng. *qâv-e penǰa,* Kal. (Tāǰ.) *qâb-e penǰar,* Gorg. *qâb penǰa*, Nud. *qâv penǰa*, etc.

4.5. It has been stated above (§ 3.4) that Kurm. Kurdish has two terms for 'finger': *tilî* and *pêçî.* If and how these two terms differ in their semantic content is not clear; the data provided by different dictionaries do not coincide completely. RIZGAR (1993) gives *tilî* (also *ṯilîk*) as 'finger' and 'toe' and *pêçî* as 'toe' and 'finger'. He also lists s.v. *tilî* the names of the individual fingers (all designations containing the word *tilî*) and s.v. *pêçî* the names of the individual toes (all designations containing the word *pêçî*). From this fact alone, one would deduce that in Kurm. Kurdish, fingers and toes are distinct lexically, or at least, that there are distinct items basically meaning either 'finger' or 'toe', which, according to the context, may be opportunely determined by *desṯ* 'hand' or *p̱ê* 'feet'. KURDOEV (1960) agrees with RIZGAR (1993) as far as *tilî* is concerned, but *pêçî* is simply glossed 'digit [*palec*]'. Similarly CHYET 2003 has *bêç'î* (also *bîçî, pêç'î, pîçî*) 'finger, toe; fingertip', given as a synonym of *tilî.* In OMAR 1992 *pîç* 'Finger' (*pîçî* 'Fingerspitze') contrasts with *bêçî* 'Zehe'; in AMÎRXAN 1992 *pîç* is 'Finger'; in LUCERI 2004 *tilî* is 'dito della mano' and *pêçî* 'dito del piede'. However it is, should really exist a stable lexical differentiation in some Krd. areas between FINGER and TOE, there is no doubt that this has to be considered as a secondary, very recent differentiation, possibly justified by the linguistic pressure exerted on the Kurdish emigrants abroad by the languages of their new homelands.[122]

As for SouthKrd. dictionaries, SAFIZĀDE 2001 gives *pîçî* as 'finger (of the hand)' while in HAŽĀR 1990, *pîčî* is recorded as 'the last joint of a finger'. ADIB TUSI 1963–1964 has an entry *poččak* 'digit [*angošt*]' attributed to Kurdish.

---

[121] For Prs. *qāb*, one cannot exclude some blending with Prs. *ka^{c}b* 'anklebone' (< Ar.).

[122] See also above, p. 48. One cannot exclude that the association of *pêçî* to 'toe', seemingly operated by lexicographers, may have been influenced by the initial *pê°*, which matches with *pê* 'foot'.

To Krd. *pêçî/bêçî* belongs Zā. *bečik* 'finger' (*bēcak(a)* in Vahman – Asatrian 1990) and probably also Māz. (Kelār.) *meček* 'finger'. Paul (1998: 212) points out that Zā. *bečik* is a lexical feature of the Alevi dialectal area, as opposed to *gišt*, marking the Çermik-Siverek and Palu-Bingöl dialectal areas.

There is a Phl. word on which we should dwell a little. It is written <bck'>, a writing which implies at least two possible transcriptions, <c> being used for phonemic /č/ or /z/. The graphic ambiguity has given rise to the contrasting stances taken up by Williams (1990-I: 206–207, 1990-II: 97) and Kotwal – Kreyenbroek (1995: 74–75) in reading two passages from the *Pahlavi Rivāyat accompanying the Dādestān ī Dēnīg* and *Nērangistān* respectively, which convey almost identical contents: both give directions on the correct way to perform the Drōn cerimony. *PRDd.* 58.26 and *Nēr.* 10.47 describe the proper way in which the *barsom* should be held: one should take it from the right hand and place it in the left; one should not hold it raised or lowered; one should hold it forwards and «APš bck' QDM BYN HNHTWNšn'». Williams' transcription and translation of the passage is as follows: *u-š bazag abar andar nihišn* "and one should hold it above sin[?]". Differently, Kotwal – Kreyenbroek transcribe and translate: *u-š bačag abar andar nihišn* "and extend one's fingers over it". This was also the interpretation of the relevant *PRDd.* passage by Jamasp-Asa (1985: 341, 348; *u-š bačak apar andar nihišn* "and one shall place his fingers on it").

Although Williams' statement (1990-II: 253) that «*bazag* "sin, evil" seems as likely a reading of MSS *bck'* as J-A's *bačak* "fingers" or G-G's **čang*»[123] cannot be challenged in theory, it is indisputable that here the meaning 'sin' appears not consistent (as Williams himself seems to be aware of, putting a question mark at the end of his translation of 58.26). Questioning Williams' interpretation, Kotwal – Kreyenbroek (1995: 75 fn. 205) read <bck'> as *bačag* 'finger', referring it to the form *bačag* used as a linear measure, and already known in the previous literature.

Phl. *bačag* (alternative spelling <bwck'>; cf. *bochak, bûchak* Kapadia 1953: 312, 325) occurs as 'joint of a finger'; see e.g. the passage where instructions are given on the correct treatment of fingernail parings (*Vd.* 17, 7, Anklesaria 1949: 343), to be buried in a pit "as much deep as the top-most

[123] Williams 1990 uses J-A and G-G as the abbreviations for Jamasp-Asa 1985 and for an unpublished transcription and translation of *PRDd.* 58 by Ph. Gignoux and F. Grenet. However, Frantz Grenet has recently informed me that the two authors do not mantain any more their previous interpretation of this passage.

joint of the smallest finger [*kehist angust frāzdōm bačag*]". It is also used as a short linear measure (2 fingers breadth; = Gr. *κόνδυλος*; HENNING 1942: 235).

Phl. *bačag* translates YAv. *t̰biši-* 'finger joint' as well as YAv. *baši-* (*FrO.*, Ch. XVI: 'ein Längenmass', BARTHOLOMAE 1904; '2 fingers breadth', HENNING 1942: 235) occurring in *Nēr.* 108 (WAAG 1941: 106) in the YAv. compound *baši-draǰaŋhō*. The interpretation of *baši-* in the *FrO.* remains doubtful: *baši-* is inserted in a list of words starting with *b-* and not semantically arranged. On account of the Phl. gloss <bcynk>, JAMASPJI – HAUG (1867) suggested 'cucumber'. REICHELT (1901: 152) identified the word as the Av. *baši-* already found in *Nēr.*; however, he provided no explanation for its Phl. counterpart. According to HENNING (ibid.: fn. 6), one should consider Av. *t̰biši-* and *baši-* as «mere spelling of the same word». To accept HENNING's suggestion, however, one should assume that the spelling *t̰b-* (alternating with *b-*) could have developed "bizarrement", as it was for *t̰kaēša-* < **kaiša-* (KELLENS 1989: 41), and not as the regular outcome of an original **du̯-* (as Gath. *daibiš* : YAv. *t̰biš* = Ved. *dviṣ*). Alternatively, one could assume that the *b*-forms have derived from a "réfection', as suggested by TREMBLAY (2005: 180), who connects here Wan. *wuzay* 'petit empan (écartment entre le pouce et l'index)' («pehl. *bck* **bazag* 'condyle, phalange' < **bazaka-*, probablement une réfection de *(*d*)*bazah-* < *d^{h}b^{h}énĝ^{h}·os, *d^{h}b^{h}n̥ĝ^{h}·és-os, cf. av. réc. *baṣi.drāǰanhō* N.108; cité *baši* F. 16, *t̰bišiš* V.6,10 [...] < *d^{h}b^{h}n̥ĝ^{h}·s-i-, πάχος 'épaisseur'»).

HENNING's suggestion has been rejected by SCHWARTZ (*apud* CHYET 2003 s.v. *bêç'î*), according to whom the «Pahl form, probably /bač(č)ak/, and the Kurdish form as well, likely represent diminutive formations in *-č-* to *baši-*», while «Av. *t̰biši-* (glossed by Pahl *bck*) 'joint (of a finger)' should be a different word, since it cannot be reconciled phonically with the group *baši-*/*bck*/bêç'î. The form *t̰biši-* would be from ProtoIE **du̯is* = 'twice, in two' (Av. *biž-uuat̰-*); the notion of 'joint' being bifurcation».

One could also assume that Av. *baši-* (and *t̰biši-*?) is in fact not Avestan. Could it be a MPrs. word in Av. garb? I do not think so, given the small number of occurrences of *bačag* in Phl. texts and the nature of the texts in which it occurs. These Av. and Phl. forms could witness the existence of some similar word(s) denoting '(part of) finger', and consequently used as a linear measure in some language(s) probably spoken somewhere in the WIr.

area. Modern outcomes would be Krd. *pêçî/bêçî*, Zā. *bečik* 'finger' and Bast. *angošt bačo,* Farām. *boča, bača* 'thumb' (see also below, p. 117).[124]

What is the motivation underlying Krd. *pêçî/ bêçî* etc.? The immediate preceding step could be a metonymical association KNUCKLE → FINGER, but the conceptualization path which has produced the word for 'knuckle' remains unclear.

5. Fingers are undoubtedly body elements of small dimension. This obvious realization is responsible for a few Ir. words for 'finger'.

Since adjectives for 'small' are often used as nominals in the sense of 'small child', when we analyse terms for 'finger' or the names of individual fingers derived from, or related to a term meaning 'small', it is often difficult to state if the conceptual pattern involved in the denominative process is (1) the plain acknowledgement of a physical dimension; (2) a CHILD = FINGER equating process, like that which could be behind EBal. *čukī*, a derivative from *čuk* 'child' meaning 'finger' according to MAYER (1910 s.v.) and GILBERTSON (1925 S.V.).[125] We will repeatedly be faced with this problem in what follows. Here I will quote Xor. (Qā, Box.) *līlī* 'finger' (also 'small; small child'; ŠĀLČI 1991) and Taj. *lela, lelak, lelik* 'finger' (*lelak, lelik* marked as "colloquial" in RAHIMI – USPENSKAJA 1954). EBal. *kūko*, 'finger' in MAYER 1910 and 'little finger' in HETU-RAM – DOUIE 1898, could be explained in this perspective as well; for further details see below p. 173.

Xor. *līlī* and Taj. *lela* are the result of a syllabic reduplication process, a lexical device with an ideophonic value, much productive in Iranian. As further instances of the *lVlV*-type, evoking the idea of smallness, one may quote Kerm. *lelu* 'a small thing', *lelânu* 'very small (mostly said of little and meagre children)' (ANJOM ŠOᶜĀᶜ 2002), Zar. *lilu* 'very little', Sirǰ. *lilāsku* 'meagre and thin', Bard. *lilaasku* 'very small', Jir.-Kahn. *lolûsk* 'small', *lal* 'small of birds or animals', Zarq. *lili* 'small (also used as an endearing term for children)', Avarz. *līla* 'baby' (ADIB TUSI 1963–1964), etc. A different explanation has been advanced by MONCHI-ZADEH (1990: no. 308), who connects Xor. *līlī* 'finger' to Xor. *klīk* 'id.', «mit Reduplikation und Ausfall beider *k*».

---

124 Note also Tāl. *biǰə, buǰə, piǰə* 'hollow of the hand; handful' and Khwar. *pck, bck* 'palm of the hand'. Is it possible to envisage any connections of these latter words with our words for '(part of) finger'?

125 On Bal. *čukī* 'little finger' see below, p. 152.

Similarly, one may consider *čimčiloq, čimčaloq* 'finger' used in (Taj.) Jugi[126], as an instance of a *č*V*č*V-pattern. Taj. speakers from Samarqand also use *čimčilok* 'finger' and MIRZOZODA (2008) records *činčilik* as a Yγn. alternative for 'finger' (but is 'little finger' in ANDREEV – PEŠČEREVA 1957). For further comments on *čimčilok* see below, p. 172.

SMALLNESS could also have been in some way responsible for dial. Taj. *čilik* 'finger' (Prs. *čelk* 'little finger') and the *kelk*-type group, for which different proposals have been advanced above, p. 65 and 63.

6. The universal attitude of human people to attribute to fingers a human nature, and perceive them as linked each other by kindred relationship, motivates the Prs. expression *dah xatani* 'the ten fingers' (DEHX with references), which depicts the fingers as *xatan*, a word (< Ar.) designating all the male relatives (father, brother etc.) of the bride. Similarly, EBal. *pādmindān* 'toes' (ELFENBEIN 1990-II) can easily be interpreted as 'the daughters of the foot', cf. EBal. *mind, minḍ* 'girl' ('bitch' elsewhere in Balochi). However, I found no confirmation of this Bal. expression in other sources and in the documentation collected in my fieldwork.

7.1. Balochi has a term for 'finger' with no equivalent in Iranian. This is *murdān*(*aγ*), also *mordān*(*aγ*), and, with metathesis, *murdaγān*. It is commonly used in EBal. varieties, but generally understood everywhere and sometimes also used in poetry by speakers of WBal./SBal. in the form of *murdān*(*ag*), perceived as a literary term. According to ELFENBEIN (1992: 252), *murdān* has spread in all Bal. dialects, at least as a measurement expression ('finger-breadth').

The etymology advanced by GEIGER (1890–1891: 242) points to the old practice of bearing seal-rings (*mur-* < *muhr* 'seal') on one's own fingers. The finger would be described as 'siegelringtragend', even if «die urspr. Bed. war offenbar ganz vergessen». The reconstructed Bal. **muhrdān* has been compared to Prs. *mohr-dār* 'keeper of the seals'. From a morphological point of view, a comparison with Bal. *zardānag* 'ring finger', i.e. the 'bearing gold finger' (see below, p. 143), reinforces GEIGER's assumption. ELFENBEIN (1990-II s.v.) points to a possible IA source, although untraced.

Note that Skt. *mudrasthāna-* denotes 'the place (on the finger) for a seal-ring'.

---

126 See above, p. 66.

7.2. Khwar. *'kwnd* 'finger' is isolated in Iranian. Possibly, it is related to *(')kwnd-* 'to beat, pound'. If so, it says something of one of the actions the finger typically performs, i.e., beating on surfaces. A similar deverbal Khwar. formation could be seen in *wyn* 'eye' from *wyn-* 'to see'.

8. Many words for 'finger' in Iranian are (more or less integrated) loans from non-Ir. languages. Some of them have been already mentioned above; cf. Prs. *qasab*, *xamse*, etc. A few others are given in the following.

Prs. *esba*ᶜ, *asba*ᶜ is a lw. from Ar. *iṣba*ᶜ; for a collection of relevant Sem. forms see MILITAREV – KOGAN 2000: no. 256. The same Sem. root (*ṢB*ᶜ) occurs in the logogram (?) accompanying Phl. *angušt* 'finger' in the *Frahang ī Pahlavīg* X, 31, reconstructed as ⁺'WS̱BᶜTH in UTAS – NYBERG 1988: 77. The Pāzand writings *hučatpaman*, *hōǰaptaman*, *hōčaptaman* (ORYĀN 1998: 163–164) clearly show how the Aramaic sequence was read in the Zoroastrian milieu of that time; HENNING (1958: 31 fn. 1) has reconstructed intermediate stages of a progressive alteration of the Aram. word which would have produced the 'fanciful' writing *hučatpaman*. The Pāzand spellings run into Persian traditional dictionaries, with the label 'Zand and Pāzand'; cf. *aučat pamun* 'finger, toe' in STEINGASS 1963 and DEHX (with further references).

Prs. *banān, banāne*, recorded as 'finger' and 'finger tip', is a loanword from Ar. *banān* 'finger, finger tip'.[127] As for Ar. *banān*, cf. Akk. *ubānu* 'finger' and the Sem. forms collected in MILITAREV – KOGAN 2000: no. 34.

Bal. *hor* is a Br. lw. commonly used by Bal. speakers living in areas where Baloch and Brahuis live in mixed communities (Noške, FILIPPONE 2000–2003: 61; Makrān, MORGENSTIERNE 1932a: 38). The Drav. etymology of Br. *hōr* (BRAY 1934) is doubtful (DED² 561).

Oss. *k'ūx/k'ox*, both 'hand' and 'finger', is Caucasian by origin (see IESOJ for references).

Dial. Taj. *barmoq* and (Kassansai) *ilikča* 'finger' (RASTORGUEVA 1963) are both Uzbek loanwords (cf. DOERFER 1967: nos 36, 111, 112).

9. A few other terms for 'finger', whose motivation escapes my analysis, or with a doubtful status in the lexicon, will be mentioned in this final paragraph.

Krd. lexicograpers record *tipil* 'finger'. Its dialectal distribution is not clear. We find it in Kurmanji dictionaries, as CHYET 2003 (*tipil* [informant from Akrê]), OMAR 1992 (*tipil, tibilk*) and AMÎRXAN 1992 (*tipil*), but also in

---

127 See also CHEBEL 1999: 85.

HAŽĀR 1990 (*tibil, tipil, dipil* 'finger'; *tapil* 'fingerprint'). KURDOEV 1960 gives *tepil* as 'extremity of limbs'; in JABA – JUSTI 1879 *tipil, tipilk* is 'extrémités des doigts'.

Prs. lexicographers record *pilaste, filaste, bilaste* 'finger' (also 'arm; cheek'), three phonetic variants to which Taj. *pilasta* 'elephant's tusk; forearm' corresponds. This word, whose primary sense is 'ivory', has been traditionally interpreted as a lexical compound formed by *pil* 'elephant' and *aste* 'bone' (see DEHX).

Prs. *pilaste* is not a neuter designation of 'finger'; it belongs to the language of poetry and, as suggested in FF and DEHX, evokes the image of 'long, white fingers', or any other parts of the body, such as the forearm or the cheeks, whose whiteness favours a mental association with ivory.[128]

I have nothing to suggest as regards Prs. *aštu, oštu* 'finger', recorded in traditional dictionaries (but not in use in Modern Prs.); Prs. *qavāre* 'fingers of the hand' (DEHX, FF), 'finger' (STEINGASS 1963); Prs. *serešt* 'toe' (STEINGASS 1963); Haz. *åxo* 'finger' (lw.?).

Khot. *hoṣ́ą̈* occurs in a later text (*Siddhasārā*) in correspondence with Buddh. Skt. *aṅgúli-* and Tib. *sor* 'finger'. The passages quoted by BAILEY (1979 s.v.) only confirm that it could be used as a linear measure. BAILEY suggests interpreting it as a 'pointed limb' (an original **fra-vaśya-* from **vaxš-* 'be pointed'). It could also be possible that this Khot. word, differently from Skt. *aṅgúli-* and Tib. *sor*, was not primarily a body part term, and had nothing to do with fingers.

Bal. *mat* 'finger' in MAYER 1910 is questionable and probably a misprint; cf. Bal. *mātī* 'thumb' below, p. 114.

128 That "whiteness" is considered as one of the forearm's salient features is also proved by the frequent association of this body part with silver or crystal in the Persian classical poetry; cf. ANUŠE 1997: 155.

CHAPTER THREE: THE THUMB

1. If it is true that the fingers are different from each other, the thumb is surely the 'most different' among them. It is felt so different that even its being a finger has been challenged.

On this point, conflicting evidence is noticeable. Gr. ἀντίχειρ (sc. δάκτυλος) 'thumb' describes this finger as being *opposite to* the fingers. The definition of Engl. *finger* in the *Oxford Dictionary of English*, second edition (2003), reads as follows: «each of the four slender jointed parts attached to either hand (or five, if the thumb is included)».[129]

How many fingers Prs. speakers instinctively attribute to hands is made clear from the mere fact that *panǰe* 'hand; the five fingers' is a derivative from *panǰ* 'five'.[130] However, there is enough evidence that Prs. speakers may also perceive and verbalize the four fingers from the forefinger to the little finger as a separate and independent concept.[131]

2. Prs. *šast*, a highly polysemic word with a wide semantic range, is the usual Prs. name of the thumb. No antecedent is recorded in Old and Middle Iranian. A quick glance at the different Prs. dictionaries shows that *šast* means: (1) '60'; (2) 'thumb (and big toe)'; (3) 'bone-ring, worn by the archers on the thumb (synonym of *zehgir*)'; (4) 'ringlets or objects with circular or semicircular shape (of rope, hair, etc.; also the sacred belt worn in the Zoroastrian rituals, more commonly called *zonnār*)'; (5) 'fish hook'; (6) 'snare, net'; (7) 'plectrum (for musical instruments)'; (8) 'string (for musical instruments)'; (9) 'lancet for phlebotomy', etc. Many of these senses are clearly related to each other. If all of them are related is not so clear. Possibly, more than one lexeme *šast* is involved: at least two homonyms could be envisaged. FF e.g. contains three different entries *šast*.

As far as I know, the origin of Prs. *šast* has not been convincingly explained.[132] We do not know whether this was a basic term for 'thumb' or originally denoted something else, with the meaning 'thumb' acquired through a

---

129 See also the definition of *finger* in COD, quoted above, p. 53, fn. 31.

130 See above, pp. 76 ff.

131 See also above, p. 42.

132 See also MOKRI 2005: 263. Ilya GERSHEVITCH, who very kindly read a draft of my paper on the finger denominations in Balochi, told me he had in mind a proposal for the etymology of *šast*, which he was still refining. I gave me no anticipation on the details on that occasion.

semantic shift, on the basis of some conceptual association. Consequently, we do not know which, if any, among the thumb's peculiar features, are highlighted with it. A few, preliminary remarks are in FILIPPONE 2000–2003: 61–62. POTT 1847: 225, fn. * emphasizes the close link between this finger and the art of practising archery.

Since an open hand in a vertical position presents four fingers standing up and one lying down (the thumb), one solution could be considering *šast* as the result of a conversion and a semantic change (through conceptual contiguity) of the past participle of (MPrs.) *šastan* 'to lie down, prostrate' (NYBERG 1974).[133] Following BAILEY's reasoning, NYBERG (ibid., with literature) points to a derivation of Phl. *šastan* from **xšata-* 'lowered'. I prefer considering Phl. *šastan* as related (same verbal root with no prefix) to MPrs. *nišastan*, Prs. *nešastan* 'to sit, sit down', for which see CHEUNG 2007: 125–126, **had* 'to sit, be seated'. Outcomes of this root with no prefix are still in use in Fārs: cf. Nud. *ša:san*, Somγ. *šasseδan*, Gorgn. *ša:siδan* (SALĀMI 2005: 254–255), Mās. *ša:seδan*, Kuz. *ša:san* (SALĀMI 2004: 252–253), Bi-rov., Dorun. *ša:seδan*, Dādenǰ. *ša:san* (SALĀMI 2006: 272–273). All of them are equivalent in meaning to Prs. *nešastan*.

Prs. *šast* 'thumb' is a current word almost everywhere in the Prs. speaking areas: cf. Taj. *šast*, Fārsivān dial. of Turkmenistan *šast* (MAHMUDOV 2001: 47), Badaxš. *šast*, Sist. *šas* (AFŠĀR SISTĀNI 1986), Birǰ. *šas*(*t*). Bal. *šast* 'thumb' represents a lexical feature of the WBal. areas, where it is very likely a Prs. loanword. Prs. loanwords are also Par. *šast* (*γušt*) (IIFL-I) and Sgl. *šast-iŋgit*.

Prs. *šast* and its cognates (or simply Prs. loans) are also found in the following dialectal areas: (1) Central/SouthKrd. dialects; cf. Sul. *emust y shest*, Krmnš. *šas*;[134] (2) the Lori cluster; cf. Lo. (Xorramābād) *šas* (HASURI 1964: 24), Bxt. (ČLang) *šas*; (3) Lārestāni and Banderi; cf. Lār. *šast* (KAMIOKA – YAMADA 1979), Min. *šast*; (4) Central dialects; cf. Yzd. *engošt-i šast* (SORUŠIĀN 1956), Esf-JPrs. *šaθ*, Gz. *šās* (*šoss* ŽUKOVSKIJ 1922: 110), Xur. *šas* (FARAHVAŠI 1976: 2), Siv. *šäse* (from Andreas; *šas* LECOQ 1979), Voniš. *šost*, Zefr. *šoss*, Keš. *šoss*, Nat. *šass*, Bohr. *šast*, Sed. *šoss*, Del. *šās-dae*, Kah. *šast*, Kerm. *šast*, Abiā. *šas*, Nāi. *šas* (LECOQ 2002), Biz. *šaxs*, Ardest. *šas*, Qohr. *šas*, Tār. *šos*; (5) NWIr. area; cf. IrĀz. *šasd* (NAVĀBI 1992), Semn. *šast*(*a*), Sang. *šast*, Lāsg. *šast*, Māz. (Kelār.) *šas*.

---

133 See also Phl. *šast* 'drooping' (NYBERG 1974).

134 JABA – JUSTI 1879 has *šest* 'main' (from PALLAS 1786), which has surely originated from a misunderstanding.

The *šast*-type seems extraneous to the lexicon of the Fārs dialects; see however the isolated Dorun. *penǰe-y ša:s* 'thumb'.

3. The large size of the thumb is a universal physical feature, shared by all human beings: describing it as "the big (or strong) finger" is quite natural, and for this reason the thumb is named in many languages by means of lexicalized phrases containing basic terms for 'finger' plus adjectives meaning 'big, bulky, stout, etc.'[135]

In Iranian, many labels for 'thumb' portray it as a big finger or the biggest among the fingers. However, since many of the Ir. adjectives meaning 'big, large, stout' (with reference to physical appearance) are also used in the meaning of 'old, elder; adult' (with reference to age), or 'great, eminent, important' (with reference to social status), most of the expressions we are going to consider may be differently interpreted: one has to decide whether considering them as simply descriptive names, or as figurative ones, with the fingers equated to a human being. In this case, the thumb is singled out for its stoutness as "the eldest" or "the senior" among the fingers. To take a position in this regard is not easy. For this reason, all the "big fingers", the "old fingers", the "great fingers" etc. are gathered in this paragraph, without proceeding with a more refined sorting. The iconomastic patterns on which these denominations for 'thumb' rest are felt so "natural" and universal that they do not require further comments. In what follows (§§3.1–3.16), I will rather concentrate on the Iranian adjectives used in this connection and try to outline, when possible, their areas of diffusion.

Since some of the adjectives we are going to survey mean in a general sense 'having a large size', and are neutral with regard to the dimension considered, they may also be used to stress specific physical peculiarities, such as TALLNESS. It follows that a few "big-finger" labels are also used to name the middle finger, as it happens, e.g., to Prs. *angošt-e bozorg*.[136]

3.1. BARTHOLOMAE (1904, s.v. *maδəma-*) quotes the following Av. expressions: *kasištahe ərəzvō* [...] *maδəmahe ərəzvō* [...] *mazištahe ərəzvō* (*Vd.* 6.10–14), and translates the three genitives as "des kleinesten [...] eines mittelgrossen [...] des grössten Fingers". Correspondingly, the Phl. translation of

[135] See for instance VEENKER 1981: 368; ZVELEBIL 1985: 664 (for the Nilgiri tribal languages, Drav. family). One might produce countless examples of this naming process.

[136] For the conceptual mapping THUMB = MIDDLE FINGER (including lexical alternation), see also abov, p. 47 and below p. 139.

this passage reads: *kehist* (<ksyst>) *angust* [...] *miyānag angust* [...] *mehist* (<msyst>) *angust*. ANKLESARIA (1949: 136–137) translates: "of the smallest finger [...] of the middle (medium) finger [...] of the biggest finger".

BARTHOLOMAE's and ANKLESARIA's interpretations are fully motivated by a rhetoric figure recurrent in Av. and Phl. texts, consisting of a comparison in a highly codified manner of different elements having progressively descending or ascending dimensions. For example, in *GrBd.* II.18, the movements of the Sun, the Moon and the Stars are compared to the movement of a very large, an average-sized and a small arrow, respectively shot by a very big man by means of a very large bow, by an average-sized man by means of an average-sized bow, by a short man by means of a small bow. This *GrBd.* passage reminds the structure of the Av./Phl. *Vd.* one quoted above. Here, three different bones with different dimensions are taken into account, and their dimensions are equated to the foremost joints of three fingers, progressively bigger. However, in the case of *Vd.*, two different strategies might have coincided. I mean, it could be possible that the three mentioned adjectives on which this Av. and Phl. rhetoric figure is built, are the same used (also in the superlative)[137] in descriptive labels for individual fingers, and in particular, the thumb, the middle and the little finger. They really happen to be conceived as the 'big(gest)', the 'middle'[138] and the 'small(est)' finger. A gloss in Phl. *Vd.* 8.71 (ANKLESARIA 1949: 214) explains that, in order to expel the Druj Nasu out of the body, the left toes should be besprinkled "from the little to the big (*az keh* <ks> *tā ō meh* <ms>)". Another explanatory annotation added by the Pahlavi translator informs the reader that the opposite direction is also admitted (*hast ke az meh* <ms> *tā ō keh* <ks> *gūyēd* "there is who says from the big to the small"). Phl. *meh* (*angust*), *keh* (*angust*) should refer to, and be the name of the thumb and the little finger, respectively.

That *kasištahe ərəzvō* [...] *maδəmahe ərəzvō* [...] *mazištahe ərəzvō* could represent the gen. forms of the Av. names of three specific fingers has already been hinted at by some Avesta scholars, including some from the Zoroastrian milieu. DARMESTETER's interpretation («of the little finger [...] of

[137] Superlative forms in finger names are also found in Sanskrit; cf. *madhyamá-* 'middlemost' (RV) (CDIAL 9810); 'the middle finger'; *kaniṣṭhá-* 'youngest' (RV), 'younger brother' (Lex.) (CDIAL 2718); *kaniṣṭhā-* 'little finger' (CDIAL 2719). See also "kučektarin angošt-e dast", Prs. gloss to Yzd. *angošt-e kiliči* 'little finger' in AFŠĀR 1989.

[138] According to this interpretation, Av. *maδəma-* ('der in der Mitte befindliche, mittlere nach Lage, Reihe, Grösse, Zahl, Wert') does not entail here an intermediate stage in a scale of value, but specifically refers to a spatial collocation in the sequence of the five fingers.

the fore-finger [...] of the middle finger», 1880: 67–68) is particularly remarkable: he also thinks of three specific fingers, but not of the same fingers suggested here. While *mazištahe ərəzvō* could actually denote the middle finger, *maδəmahe ərəzvō* for the forefinger remains unmotivated.

The Buddhist Sgd. text P 14 (ll. 17–37) contains the description of a *mudrā*. Unfortunately, the text is in a very poor condition and its many gaps do not allow a good understanding of the passage. In l. 25, however, one distinctly reads *dwa mazēx angušt* (<'δw mz'yγ 'nkwšt >), which probably refers to thumbs. BENVENISTE (1940: 138) translates «les deux grands doigts». In the same passage, the names of the forefinger (*niwēδēne-angušt*) and the middle finger (*miδānč angušt*) also occur; see below p. 123 and pp. 133, 136.

Sgd. *mazēx angušt* (<mz-'yγ 'n(k)[wšt]>) also appears in the body parts list (*Book of the Limbs*) published in SUNDERMANN 2002: 142-144. In this text, however, as SUNDERMAN rightly suggests (ibid.: fn. 71), the mentioned "big finger" should be identified as the middle finger, since the name of the thumb probably occurs two lines below as *n(r)šk*.[139] It follows that the same label was used in Sogdian to refer to both the thumb and the middle finger, according to a usual practice, for which see above (p. 95). Contextual or cotextual parameters may intervene in these cases to remove any ambiguity.

As (close) parallels to Av. (gen.) *mazištahe ərəzvō* and Sgd. *mazēx angušt* 'thumb' one may quote KurmKrd. *tilîya mezin* and W/SBal. (Nal; Noške; Makrāni MORGENSTIERNE 1932a: 40) *mazanẽ lankuk,* Korš. *mazzanun penǰa*, SBal. *mastarẽ lankuk*, the latter with the comparative degree of the same adjective. These descriptive Bal. expressions may coexist with other labels for 'thumb' in the lexical repertoire of a single Bal. speaker.[140]

Av. *maz-* 'big; great, eminent', (YAv.) *mazant-* 'big, large; high' (comp. *mazya-*, sup. *mazišta-*), Sgd. *mazēx* 'great' (comp. *mazyātar*), Krd. *mazin/mezin*, Bal. *mazan* 'big, great, etc.' are commonly related to IE **meĝh-*, to which should also belong Man. MPrs. *mazan* 'monstrous; giant, monster', Khot. *maysirka-* 'large, great', Vfs. *mæzæn* 'big, large', Pšt. *mə́zay, mázay* 'big, massive, fat; strong', Wan. *múza* 'strong', as well as Skt. *mahā̃nt-* with its modern IA outcomes (EWA II: 337; CDIAL 9946).

Phl. *mahist* (<msst>) in the phrase *mahist angust*, translating Av. (gen.) *mazištahe ərəzvō* in *Vd.*, is a superlative form from *meh* (<ms>) 'great(er), old(er)'.

---

139 See below, p. 112.

140 The Bal. speaker living in Oman, for example, who provided me with *mastarẽ lankuk* 'thumb', considered it as an alternative to *mātak*.

Phl. *meh, mahist* (Man. MPrs. *mahy* 'bigger', *mahist* 'greatest, eldest') are generally referred to IE **maḱ*-, together with Av. *mas*- 'long; large, big' (comp. *masyah*-),[141] OPrs. *maθišta*- 'greatest', Man. Prth. *masišt* greatest, highest', *masādar* 'greater, older, of higher rank', Sgd. *masyātar* 'greater, higher'.

Prs. *meh* 'great', *mehin* 'greatest, eldest' continue the MPrs. *meh*-series but they are quite peripheral in the Prs. lexicon. In Modern Ir. languages, the *mas*-type[142] for 'big, etc.' characterizes the dialects of Northern and Central Iran. One may quote Semn., Lāsg. *masin*, Srx. *mosin*, Sang. *master* (sup. *masterīn*, ŽUKOVSKIJ 1922: 130), Aft. *masin*, Ham-JPrs. *mäsär* ('great'), Mah. *masar*, Āmor. *masdar* ('big', *masdatar* 'bigger'), Āšt. *masdar*, Kah. *masdar,* Anār. *masa*, Nāi. *mas, masa,* Sed. *mehīn*, Xuns. *mossar* (also *missär* in EILERS 1976), Voniš. *mussar*, Yzd-JPrs., ZorYzd., ZorKerm. (MAZDĀPUR 1995 s.v. *bozorg*) *mas*, all meaning 'big, large, great, etc.'.[143] SBšk. (Garu) *mohok* 'big' (G. BARBERA p.c.) could belong here.

As for EIr., one may mention Pšt *mə́šar, məšr* (Wan. *míser*) 'elder (brother, etc.)', referring to both age and social position (PSTRUSIŃSKA 1985–1986: 13).

It seems likely that in some areas and/or different ages, forms originally belonging to the *mas*- and the *maz*-type have merged.

3.2. Prs. *angošt-e bozorg* (Taj. *angušt-i buzurg*) is a common thumb name, alternative to *šast*. As already stated above, it may also be used to name the middle finger.

Prs. *bozorg* is the most usual Prs. term for 'big'. It covers many senses, being used with reference to real dimensional evaluation ('big, large, stout, etc.'), age ('grown, adult'), high social status ('important, eminent'), etc. In AfγPrs., however, *bɔzɔrg* is perceived by speakers as a word belonging to the classical heritage, and is actually not used for physical dimensions ('grand au sens figuré, majestueux, respectable; sage, saint, sainte', BAU 2003). The same is true for Taj. *buzurg*.

Antecedents of Prs. *bozorg* are OPrs. *vazr̥ka*- and MPrs./Prth. *wuzurg* (Paz. *guzurg*) 'big, great'. An EIr. cognate is Sgd. *wazark* (<wz'rk, wzrk>) 'big, great'. Related forms in Modern Iranian (in some cases adapted Prs. loanwords)

141 In *Vd.* 6.14 the mss. alternate between *mazišta*- and *masišta*-. This passage would be the only evidence for an Av. *mas*-form. According to R. SCHMITT (p.c.), one might assume *mazišta*- as the "correct" reading, and delete *masišta*- from the Av. documentation.

142 Comparative forms of this type are sometimes positive in meaning. A few comments on old comparatives in Xunsāri, used as positive adjectives, are in EILERS 1976: 54.

143 The *mas*-type 'big, large' is only found in the SE and NW subgroups of Central dialects; see KRAHNKE 1976: 215–217 (with Map V – 28).

are found in a few Central dialects; cf. Qohr. *bözörg* 'great', Bard. *gohark* 'big, huge', Esf-JPrs. *boδorg*, Kuhp. *vəzark* (KRAHNKE 1976: 217), etc.

To explain Kerm. *gohort*, Soi *gurt*, Farizandi *gōrd*, Bšk. *gohort* 'big', GERSHEVITCH (1964b: 12–13, fn. 4) reconstructs OP **vaδr̥ta-*, synonymous with *vazr̥ka-*, whose suffix should have been lost in Yzd. *gohor*, and in the side-forms with *-z-*, namely Bšk. *gozer* and Xur. (comp.) *girzotor*. To these latter, one may add Jir.-Kahn. *gozer*, Frv. *gazar*, and Xur. *gozår*. To a hypothetical Old SW form **vadrak(a)* > **vard(ak)* > *gurd* also points STILO (2007: 108) to explain the *gord*-type forms for 'big, large' of the Kāšān area, like Soi *gurt*, Fariz. *gōrd*, mentioned above. It could also be possible, however, that this latter group does not belong here; for a different suggestion see below, § 3.7.

3.3. Prs. *angošt-e sotorg* 'thumb' parallels Ydɣ. ^{u}*sturo-guščo* 'thumb'.

Prs. *sotorg* (a literary term, according to LAZARD 1990a), Taj. *suturg, siturg* 'large, big' have MPrs. *sturg* 'gross, coarse' as their immediate antecedent. They belong, together with Ydɣ. ^{u}*stur*, to the large IIr. lexical family which includes, in Iranian (< **stūra(ka)-*), Khot. *stura-* 'large', Bactr. αστοργο, στορογο, στοργο 'great' (SIMS-WILLIAMS 2000), Oss. *styr* (D *stur, ästur, istur, ustur*) 'big, great', Bal. (probably only EBal.) *istūr* 'coarse, thick', SouthKrd. *estûr, stûr*, KurmKrd. *stûr* 'thick, stout', Pšt. *stər* 'big, large', Ōrm. ^{u}*stur, stur*, Ydɣ. ^{u}*stur*, Mnǰ. *stur* 'big', Par. *ostāṛo, ostāṛu* 'stout, thick', etc., and, in IA, Skt. *sthūrá-, sthūlá-* 'thick, strong, etc.' (EWA II: 768–769) and its outcomes in modern IA. Possibly, here also belongs YAv. °*stūra-*, extrapolated by MAYRHOFER (1979: [78], [240]) from the proper names *Pairištūra-* and *Baēšatastūra-*.

3.4. MOKRI (2005: 263) records Prs. *angošt-e setabr* 'thumb'.

Prs. *setabr* (Taj. *sitabr*), directly following Phl. *stabr* 'big, coarse, strong', Man. MPrs. *istabr* 'strong, firm',[144] belongs to the Ir. family of Av. *staβra-*, Khot. *staura-* 'firm, strict, severe', etc., and, with a different semantic specialization, Oss. *st'ælf* (Dig. *(æ)st'ælfæ, st'ælfæg*) 'stain, point'.

[144] According to BELARDI (2009: 159), Arm. *stowar* 'coarse, big, strong' should not be considered as a "pure Armenian" word, as in HÜBSCHMANN 1897: 493, where this form is connected to the etymological family of Skt. *sthūra-*, Bal. *istūr*, etc. (see § 3.3 above), but as a loanword from Prth. *istabr*. Note, however, that the form ^{c}*stbr* referred to by BELARDI could be a MPrs. word in a Man.Prth. text (see DURKIN-MEISTERERNST 2004 s.v.).

3.5. Bxt. *kelič-e* (or *angost-e*) *gapp* (my own data), Mamas. *k̂elič-e gapu*, Knd., Hay. *penǰe-y gapu* and Lārest. (Lār., Ger.) *kelike-gapû*, all meaning 'thumb', contain *gap*-forms for 'big', characterizing a band stretching all across the region from South-Central Kurdish, Lori and Fārs areas down to the belt along the Persian Gulf in South Iran. Here belong SouthKrd. *gap* 'thick, huge', Krmnš. *gap*, SulKrd. *gep* 'bulky', Šušt. *gap,* Dezf. *gap* (comp. *gaftar*), Bxt. *gap, gaf,* (ČLang) *gap*, Mamas. *gapu*, Lo. *gap*, Šir./Kāz. *gap* 'big', Mās. *gäp* ('groß, erwachsen', Mann 1909), Zarq. *gap,* Buš. *gap*, Dašt. *gap*, Lir.-Dayl. *gap* (Lirāvi 2001: 239), Kumz. *gayp*, Min. *gap*, Horm. *gäp*, Fin. *gap*, Bast., Farām. *gap*, Xonj. and Lār. *gap* (Kamioka – Rahbar – Hamidi 1986), etc. 'big'. Apparently isolated in Central Iran we find Sirǰ. *gap* 'big and huge'. Prs. *gap/gab* 'thick', recorded in traditional dictionaries (see Dehx), should be considered as a dialectal form.

At the present state of our knowledge, the origin of this lexical set is unknown. Vahman – Asatrian (1987: s.v. *gyap*) refer to Sgd. *γarf* (<γrß/f>) 'much', but the etymology proposed for this Sgd. word by Sims-Williams (1983: 49; < **faruwam*), if accepted, would render such a connection untenable.

In fact, a form which may hardly be kept apart from Sgd. *γarf* is Buš. *γarp* 'big; notable, great; fat; aloud', *γarpele* 'abnormally big (also derogatory)'. To Sgd. *γarf,* Morgenstierne doubtfully connects Wx. *γafč* (*γafči* in IIFL-II) 'much', on which see now Steblin-Kamenskij 1999 s.v. *γa, γafč.* Some of the forms quoted ibid. (in particular Yγn. *γába* 'thick') could be easily associated to the *gap*-forms listed above. I would add here Yγn. *γaftar* 'more' (Mirzozoda 2008). As far as Wx. *γafč* is concerned, Steblin-Kamenskij (1999) points to a possible connection (old lw. with *č* < *c*) with Šγn. *γāfc* 'thick' (already in EVŠG), which in its turn could be considered as an adapted lw. from Taj. *γafs*. Taj. loanwords are also Mnǰ. *γafs* 'fat; thick' and Yγn. *γafs-* in *γafskama* 'with a thick neck' (Mirzozoda 2008). However, as Steblin-Kamenskij 1999 rightly underlines, the origin of Taj. *γafs* is by no means clear: it could be itself a lw. from an EIr. language. Compare also Taj. (Dušanbe) *qaws* 'gros (homme, animal)' (Bau 2003), AfγPrs. *γabs, gabz* 'large, broad-shouldered man' (Mazār-e Šarif *γafs* Bau 2003), Haz. *γʌps* 'very fat' (*γabs* Bau 2003), Madagl. *γafs*, Badaxš. *γaws* 'thick (of a stock etc.)'.

Should it be possible to prove some kind of connection between the WIr. *gap*-type and Šγn. *γāfc*, we could add Šγn. *γāfc angix̌t* 'thumb' (Zarubin 1960) to the thumb names listed at the head of this paragraph.

3.6. Dav. *pinǰe-y gotu*, Dahl., Mās., Somγ., Ban., Pāp., Dusir., Rič., Gorgn., Mosq., Kal. (Lor), Baliā., Birov., Dādenǰ. *penǰe-y gotu*, Kuz., Dežg. *penǰe-y gottu*, Kal. (Tāǰ.) *penǰar-e gat*, Siv. *gusse gutū* (ŽUKOVSKIJ 1922: 110) and Abd. *penǰe-y get* (*angušte get* ŽUKOVSKIJ 1922: 110) 'thumb', all from Fārs, induce the following considerations.

The *got*-type adjective for 'big, huge, thick' is a lexical feature of the Fārs dialectal area; cf. Šir. *got* (with particular reference to physical size), Kāz., Gavk., Sarv., Dav., Dahl., Kal. (Lor), Ban., Rič., Pāp. (also 'tall'), Dusir., Mosq., Somγ. (also 'tall'), Gorgn., Nud., Baliā., Birov., Hay., Dādenǰ., Dāreng., Dorun., Dežg., Mās., Zarq. *got*, Kuz. *guvet*, Kal. (Tāj.) *gat*, Buringuni *gut* (MANN 1909), Mamas. *got, γot* (LIRĀVI 2001: 243), *gut* (MANN 1910), Abd. *get* 'big'.

The *got*-type is also found along the coastal strip South of Fārs and eastwards up to Lārestān; compare Lir.-Dayl. *got, γot* (LIRĀVI 2001: 239, 243), Buš., Dašt., Fin., Lār., Farām., Bast. *got* 'big'.

The presence of *got* 'big' in Koroši, the Bal. dialect spoken in Fārs, is due to the influence of Fārs dialects on Koroši. The same could be true for Sivandi, generally acknowledged as a Central dialect, where one find *gut* 'big' (ZIĀN 1960), *gutū* 'big' (*gut(u/ə)kunū* 'eldest, biggest').[145] However, though not so diffused as in Fārs and South Iran, the *got*-type is not completely extraneous to Central dialects; see Ardest. *got* 'great', Sirǰ. *got* 'big and thick' (ĀZĀDIXĀH 1983).

Abd. *get* 'big' has parallels in Kurdish, as is quite natural, being Abdui a Krd. dialect spoken in Fārs; cf. SouthKrd. *git, kit* 'prominent, big', *gita* 'huge', Krmnš. *get* 'big and huge, hefty'.

Prs. lexicographers record *gote* 'great, large, grand' and *gat, gate* 'id.' (DEHX). These are with all probability dialectal items, with a specific areal connotation: while the *got*-type characterizes Fārs and South Iran, the *gat*-type seems to be mostly diffused in Māzandarān and Northern Iran. Compare Māz. *gat, gati* 'big; grandfather', Qasr. *gaht, gahte, gahta* 'big', Tehr. *gat* 'big' (ADIB TUSI 1963–1964), but also Kal. (Tāǰ.) *gat* 'big' in Fārs. In Colloquial Persian, the adjectival compound *got-o-gonde* 'big, thick (and un-

[145] EILERS (1988) dubitatively suggests a connection between Siv. *gutū* and Soi/Kalun (Kalān)-Abdui *gurd/t*. Similarly, in CHRISTENSEN – BARR 1939: 469 there is a cross-reference between Soi *gurt* and Kal.-Abd. *git*. I think that the two lexical clusters (*gord/gerd*-type and *got*-type) are not (directly) connected and should be kept apart. See also below, § 3.7.

shapely)'[146] (NAJAFI 1999) has the intensive semantic implication of the (pseudo) echo-compounds; similarly, one finds *kat-o-gonde* 'large, big' (NAJAFI 1999) and *kat-o-koloft* 'corpulent' (LAZARD 1990a). Is *kat-* a meaningless ideophonic device, or an autonomous lexical form?

In fact, *kat-* recalls a group of adjectives fairly widespread in the Eastern Ir. world, namely in Eastern Persian and EIr. languages. One may quote Sist. *kata* 'big, huge', AfγPrs. *kata* 'big', Her. *katta*, (dial) Taj. *kata, katta* 'big; adult' (RASTORGUEVA 1963, ROZENFEL'D 1982),[147] Haz. *kaṭa* 'big, large; aged, old, adult' (*katta* 'tall', Kāb. 'thick, coarse' DULLING 1973), Pšt. *kaṭá* 'big', Yγn. *kátta* 'big, large; aged, eminent', Par. *kaṭo, kato* 'old', Išk. *kata* 'big', Šγn. *kata-* 'big, elder, adult', *katā, kattā* 'big; senior; adult; experienced', Oroš. *ketā* 'groß' (LENTZ 1933), etc. Birǰ. *kotta*, which has been recorded in a 19th c. dictionary by Mollā ᶜAli Ašraf Sabuhi with the meaning of 'big', nowadays rather means 'fat and compressed' (REZĀI 1966).

Cognate forms are found in Central dialects, though not so homogenously diffused; cf. Sirǰ. *katte* and Xur. *kattå* 'big, huge'. In addition, we may mention here IrĀz. (Ker.) *ketma* 'big' (ZOKĀ 1954: 58), and a few *l*-derivatives such as Māz. (Tabari) *katal* 'huge, large' (ADIB TUSI 1963–1964), Lo. *kotil* 'huge, large' (ADIB TUSI 1963–1964), Xor. *γotol* 'fat and large; round' (see MONCHI-ZADEH 1990: 79), Yzγ. *qatol* 'big; large; adult', etc.

It has been suggested that some or all the Ir. *kata*-forms are due to the influence of Eastern Turkish languages, particularly Uzbek.[148] However, how the relevant forms in Eastern Turkish are linked to each other is by no means clear;[149] an Ir. ultimate origin is not to be excluded for them, as suggested by ORANSKIJ (1970: 158 fn. 26), who points to an OIr. base **katăna-* (Šγn. *katanak* should also belong here). Furthermore, it seems reasonable enough to associate to Pšt. *kaṭá* 'big', the *γ*-series of Pšt. *γaṭ* 'big, stout; fat; great in rank or power', Wan. *γuṭ* 'fat' and Ōrm. *γuṭ* (K. *gwaṭ*, Lo. *ghoṭa*) 'fat', even if the details are still unclear. Whatever may be the origin of the *kata*-forms

---

[146] Cf. also Buš. *got-o-gonde* 'very big' (used as a mockery term); Yzd-JPrs. *gad-o-gondo*, Hanǰ. *gat-o-gonda* 'id.'.

[147] FZT, mostly including literary Tajik, does not record *kat(t)a*, which probably only belongs to the informal/colloquial register.

[148] See for instance ANDREEV – PEŠČEREVA 1957 (for Yγn. *kátta*), MORGENSTIERNE (IIFL-II; for Išk. *kata*) and LENTZ 1933 (for Oroš. *ketā*).

[149] There are also scholars (as for example BOGDANOV mentioned by LENTZ 1933: 173), who have attempted to derive the Turk. forms from Hi. *kittā, kettā* 'how much?'. One could wonder why then not to point directly to Hi. *kaṭṭā* 'stout, strong, etc.', which, though not satisfactorily explained itself, seems hardly detachable from our *kata*-forms.

in Iranian and Central Asian languages, this lexical cluster seems to represent an areal feature with a wide diffusion.

One could even wonder whether some kind of relationship between the *kata*-group and the *got*-group mentioned above may be envisaged. A suggestion by MONCHI-ZADEH (1990: 237), who however does not take into consideration the Turkish evidence, goes in that direction. I agree with him in principle, even if all the matter requires much prudence and many phonetic details are still to be sorted out. Be that as it may, contamination and blending among the different lexical groups treated in this paragraph might easily have happened.

All this considered, we might add the following thumb names to the list at the top of this paragraph:[150] Pšt. *γaṭá gúta, kaṭá gúta*, Ōrm. *γuṭṭa-ŋgušt* (MORGENSTIERNE 1932b), Sgl. *katta narxåk* and Yγn. *katta paxxa* (MIRZOZODA 2008, s.v. *paxxa*), which is however recorded as one of the names of the forefinger as well.[151]

3.7. KurmKrd. *tilîya girdikê* (RIZGAR 1993) 'thumb' contains a derivative of Krd. *girde* 'big' (KURDOEV 1960). ŽUKOVSKIJ (1922: 110) records Siv. *šasse gird* 'thumb', a lexicalized phrase whose head itself means 'thumb'.[152] Such apparently pleonastic expressions might be a peculiarity of popular/low registers. I recorded e.g. *šast bozorg* 'thumb' from a woman, native speaker to Kermānšāh, who strongly questioned that *šast* alone (viz. not modified by *bozorg*) could be considered as an "acceptable" name for that finger.

Krd. *girde* and Zā. (Çermik) *gird* (Kiği *girs*) 'big, large' (see also HADANK 1932: 156) find their motivation in the mental association equating ROUNDNESS (cf. Prs. *gerd* 'round') with BIGNESS, according to a well known iconomastic pattern, on which Prs. *gonde* 'big' and cognates also rest.[153] I

---

[150] Thumb names in some Turk. dialects spoken in Xorāsān also contain *kata* 'big'; cf. Douγā'ī *kata birmax*, Joγatāy *kata burmax*, Jonk *kata bïrmax*, Qara-Bāγ *kata aŋguštin*, etc. (DOERFER – HESCHE 1993, pp. 106, 149, 160, 213).

[151] See below, p. 131. Cf. the Yγn. sentence *či du katta paxxaiš tirš xorta* "he got a bullet in his two big finger (= thumb and index finger were torn off by a bullet)" in MIRZOZODA 2008, s.v. *paxxa*[1].

[152] See Siv. *šas* 'thumb', quoted above, p. 94.

[153] Cf. ROSSI 2002: 155 ff. Dimensional concepts other than BIGNESS are also associated to the notion of ROUNDNESS. Words for 'round' may acquire the meaning of 'squat' or even 'small, short'; see e.g., Xor. *girdī*, SouthKrd. *gird*, *girda*, etc., Xuns. *girdilä* (EILERS 1976), Dav. *gerdel*, Zarq. *gerdelak,* Buš. *gerdele*, Bxt. (ČLang) *gerdela* (also *gerd-o-gelil*), all meaning 'plump and short person'. See also Dav. *moR-ek* 'plump and short per-

suggest associating here the *gord*-type 'big', mainly spread in Central Iran, where it characterizes a north-central dialectal sub-area (KRAHNKE 1976: 215–217, Map V-28). For a different explanation see above, § 3.2.

3.8. The adjectives for 'big' occurring in the thumb names in a few languages of the Šγn. group, in particular Šγn. *baq angix̌t*, Bart., Baǰ. *beq ⁱŋgax̌t* (SKÖLD 1936: 140), and Roš. *bēq ingax̌t,* are similarly motivated by the conceptual association ROUNDNESS = BIGNESS.

Šγn. *boq* (fem. *baq* and *beq*), Roš.-Xuf. *boq* (fem. *bēq*), etc. 'projecting; bulky; big' parallel *buγ* and *buq* 'bulky, big', found in the Taj. dialects of Darvāz and Vanǰ (ROZENFEL'D 1982), respectively. Elsewhere, cognate *buq*-forms refer to the general property of being round (Yzγ. *poq* 'round') or are used as words for specific things having a round and projecting shape, belonging to the body and landscape domains. In particular, they may denote (1) humps in human and/or animal bodies; cf. Pšt. *bok* 'hump; raising; bump', Haz. *boko* 'camel's hump', Yγn. *bŭk* 'hump; humpbacked', *bŭkra* 'humpbacked' (*buka* MIRZOZODA 2008), Taj. *bukak*, Yzγ. *poqmaδən*, Oss. *būk'* (Dig. *bok'*) 'humpbacked'; (2) hillocks, mounds, and similar natural elements; cf. Pšt. *bok*, Wx. *buq*, dial. Taj. (Darvāz, Vanǰ) *bəqi* (ROZENFEL'D 1982), Badaxš. *buq*, Sariq. (TV) *bïq*, (B) *bůq*, Roš., Xuf. *boq*, *boqay*, Yzγ. *poq*, Mnǰ. *buq*, Išk. *bïq*, Oroš. *boq*, Šγn. *buq*, etc.

AfγPrs. *buγund* 'round (thing)', *buγundī* 'hillock; mound of earth' (also 'fat baby'), Her. *boqond* 'projecting and raising thing', Haz. *buγundi* 'mound; hill' could be explained as the result of a merger of two different words (*buq* and *γund*).

The origin of these *buq*-forms is unknown; they could also be Turk. elements in Iranian, as suggested by ANDREEV – PEŠČEREVA 1957 (Yγn. *bŭk* < Uzb.) and by STEBLIN-KAMENSKIJ 1999 (Wx. *buq*, Taj. or Turk. lw.). ABAEV convincingly points to a phonosymbolic basis (IESOJ I: 269). That the *buq*-form is a lexical feature typical of the Eastern Ir. regions seems to be indisputable. However, a few traces of it can also be found in the Iranian West: cf. Jir.-Kahn. *bok* 'bulgy, prominent, embossed', Šušt. *boq* 'bubble on the water; prominence' (FĀZELI 2004).

3.9. An adjectival base for 'big' characterizes the Kurdish, Gorāni and Zāzā speaking areas. Here we find KurmKrd. *gumre, gumreh* 'big, huge; powerful'

---

son' as contrasted with *moR* 'round'; Buš. *gompulak* 'any round thing' as contrasted with *gempel* 'plump and short person', etc.

(CHYET 2003), *gewre* 'big, large' (RIZGAR 1993, KURDOEV 1960), *givr, givrik* (CABOLOV 2001), (Sul.) *gewre* 'big, grown up, senior', SouthKrd. *gawr* 'big', *gawra* 'great, aged, senior', (Mahâb.) *gawra* 'big (in a physical sense)', (Garr.) *gāorä* 'tribal chief', Gor. (Awr.) *gawra* 'big', (Kand.) *gaurä, gourä, gourî* 'great, powerful; aged, elder', (Gahw.) *gôûrä* 'great, big', (Bāǰalāni) *gaur* 'great, big; senior' (HADANK 1930: 420). Here also belongs *gôrâ* 'big' found in Koruni, a dialect of Krd. origin spoken in Fārs.

Kurdish has most likely influenced dialects spoken in the surrounding areas, namely Fārs and Lori areas, as is proved by Šušt. *gowra* 'big, stout, thick', Dav. *gavor* 'big, of robust frame', Dašt. *geverak* 'grown (said of children starting early to walk or the like)';[154] see also Šahm. *gowre* 'big'. In the Čahār Lang dialect of Baxtiāri, *gowra* has acquired the restricted sense of 'particularly big male dog'; IZADPANĀH 2001 attributes the same sense to *gowra* found in the Lori dialects of Pāpi and Bālā Garive. In the dialect of this latter village, *gur* means 'thickness, fullness' (AMANOLAHI – THACKSTON 1986).

No convincing explanation of the origin of this lexical group has been advanced so far. HADANK (1930: 250) quotes an improbable suggestion by KARST connecting it to Sumerian *guru* 'high'. CHRISTENSEN – BARR (1939: 301) tentatively point to an OIr. base **garu-*, to which they also relate Av. *gouru-* 'schwer' and Pšt. *γar-* in *γar-nīkə́* 'great grandfather' (see EVP and NEVP). CABOLOV 2001 suggests a derivation of Krd. *givr* etc. from *gumre*, which is given as a lw. from Turk. *gümrah*.

Bxt. (ČLang) *gowra* 'particularly big male dog' shows striking analogies with Sist. *bowr* 'big and bad-tempered dog'. MOHAMMADI XOMAK (2000 s.v.) considers *bowr* as the "ancient pronunciation" of Prs. *babr* 'tiger', and *sag-e bowr* as basically meaning *sag-e babrgune* 'tiger-coloured dog', adding that nowadays only few Sistāni people would be aware of this. AfγPrs. *babar* means 'hairy, shaggy', and *babrak* denotes a kind of thick, coarse woollen cloth. In the Ir. Bal. area that is largely influenced by Sistāni, however, and in particular in Sarāwāni, Lāšāri and the dialect of Gošt,[155] *bowr* is an adjective meaning 'thick'. On the occasion of an interview focussed on the dimensional domain lexicon, a Bal. speaker from Gošt used *bowr* with a very high frequency in order to describe thick pieces of wood, legs, thread and similar things (*bowrẽ dār, bowrẽ pādā̃, bowrẽ bandīk* etc.). Does Sist. *bowr* 'big dog' have really something to do with *babr* 'tiger', as suggested

[154] Cf. also the Dašt. sentence *beče-yku geverak vâvide* 'that child has grown a lot [*ān bačče nesbatan bozorg šode*]'.

[155] Information taken from an unpublished (Ir.) Bal. dictionary, for which see above, fn. 97.

by MOHAMMADI XOMAK? I would prefer looking for another solution, also in the light of forms like Zefr. *bür* 'big' (ŽUKOVSKIJ 1888: 75).[156] The whole question appears particularly entangled but it sounds intriguing, and merits a closer investigation, which I reserve for another occasion. One could also think of reassessing the case of the OIr. proper name recorded in Elamite writing as *kam-ra-ak-ka*$_4$ and *ka*$_4$*-u-ra-ak-ka*$_4$. The reconstructed OIr. form **Gauraka-* (*-ka*-extension of **Gaura-*) has been interpreted as 'wild ass' by GERSHEVITCH (the same as the MIr. proper name *Gōr*) and has been related to Old IA *ghorá-* 'inspiring fear' by MAYRHOFER (and recently also by TAVERNIER 2007: 188 and 589 with literature).

The thumb names containing the mentioned adjectives for 'big' are the following: SorKrd. *qamkî gewre* (KURDOEV – JUSUPOVA 1983), Sul. *emustegewre, pencegewre*, SouthKrd. *kilka gawra* (*angusta / kilka / panǰa gawra* SAFIZĀDE 2001, *angûsa gawra* EBRĀHIMPUR 1994a), Krmnš. *kelek gâwrâga* (besides *kelek bozorga*), Mukri *qâmîk-e gawrah*, Gor. (Gahw.) *kilik-i gôûrä*.

3.10. The adjectival base contained in Gil. *pile angušt* and Zā. *engişta pîl* (TODD 1985) 'thumb' is spread all along a north-western band, including Gilaki, some varieties of Ir. Āzari, Tāleši and Zāzā, with the meaning of 'big'. Instances are Gil. *pile* 'big; large; strong, powerful; bulky; tall', (Rāms.) *pilā, pile* 'big', IrĀz. (Šāli) *pilla*, (Hazārrudi) *pille*, (Tākestāni) *pella* (LECOQ 1989a: 304), (Sagz., Ebr.) *pila*, (Čā.) *pil(l)a*, Tāl. (Zidei, Māsāl) *pille* (BAZIN 1981: 276), Zā. *pīl* 'old; eldest; big' (Siverek, Čabaxčur *pil*, Kur *pîl* in HADANK 1932: 163), etc.

There is no satisfactory etymology for the *pil*-'big' lexical group. EILERS (1979) mentions Gil. *pil(l)e* s.v. Gz. *bäli, bälĕ* 'groß', which he refers to SW Ir. **barda-* 'hoch'. In HADANK 1932: 295, 296, Zā. (Kur) *pîl* 'alt; groß' and *pîr* 'alt' are cross-referred and both related to Prs. *pir* 'old, aged'. The same connection has been suggested in JABA – JUSTI 1879, where s.v. *pīl* 'grand, l'aîné', labelled as Zāzā, Krd. *pîr* 'vieux, viellard' is quoted. HENNING (1954: 164 fn.4), however, rejected HADANK's hint («Zaza *pîl* [...] often wrongly confused with Prs. *pīr* 'old'»), without any further comment.

Prs. *pir* 'old, aged', as well as its MPrs. antecedent *pīr* (< **par-ya-*; see GERSHEVITCH 1964a: 82), is always used with reference to social hierarchy ('head; spiritual leader') or age ('old'), and never works as a dimensional ad-

---

[156] STILO (2007: 108) suggests for Zefr. *bür(g)* a possible derivation from OIr. **vadraka-* (**vadrak(a)* > **vadark* > **vadarg* > *bu(d)arg* > *bürg*).

jective. Since the BIG → AGED transfer represents a privileged conceptual path in Iranian, the inverse process could be considered as predictable as well. A confirmation is given by Daštestāni, where *pir*, besides its usual sense of 'old', has also acquired that of 'big, large, huge' (qualifying things), as proved by phrasal expressions such as *pir čomâq* 'big cudgel', *pir sang* 'big stone', etc.

Waiting for a better explanation, I would not completely discard a Prs. *pir* ~ Zā. *pīl*, etc. connection. This could be supported by the *l* > *r* development in a few words, which at least resemble Prs. *pir* 'old', in languages of the area where the *pil*-'big' group is found. An instance is Gil. (Rāms.) *pilālsāl* 'the year before last' as contrasted with Prs. *pirārsāl* (*pirār* < **para-yār*- GERSHEVITCH 1964a: 82).

Should we somehow relate Wx. *pUluk* 'thumb' (for which MORGENSTIERNE [IIFL-II] tentatively suggests a connection with Lat. *pollex*) to Gil. *pile angušt* and Zā. *engişta pîl*?

3.11. In Southern Kurdish, we find *kilka ka<u>l</u>a*, *ka<u>l</u>a amust/angust* (*panǰ kala* SAFIZĀDE 2001), Garr. *kelik e kal*, all meaninig 'thumb'; see also Sul. *ke<u>l</u>emust*, Gor. (Talahed.) *kelek kalena* and Lak. *kel̄ekekela* .

To these Kurdish and Gorāni thumb names, the following may be associated: (1) (West Iran) Lo. *kalak-e kala* (UNVALA 1958: 15), (Xorramābād) *kelek kala* (HASURI 1964: 24); (2) (North Iran) Gil. *kale-angušt*, (Māč.) *kal angušt,* (Rāms.) *kalə ongušt*, Tāl. (Rep. of Azerbaijan) *kəllə angĭštə* (PIREJKO 1976), (Kargānrudi) *kela angəšta*, (Asālemi) *kəla angəšta* (D. GUIZZO p.c.); (3) (Central Iran) Gz. *kal*; (4) (EIr. languages) Yzγ. *kəlγ*^{w}*ax̌t, qəlγ*^{w}*ax̌t* and (comparative degree) *kəldūr wax̌t* 'thumb' (GAUTHIOT 1916: 254 fn.1), also quoted in SKÖLD 1936: 186 (*qəlduri u̯ax̌t*); ĖDEL'MAN 1971 has *qəldůri γ*^{w}*ax̌t* as 'middle finger'.

The adjectives occurring in the lexicalized phrases mentioned above belong to Prs. *kal* 'big' (DEHX; only in *kalčašm* 'big-eyed'), which is with all probability a "dialectal" form. Consider Šir. *kal* 'big', Birǰ. *kalə* 'big, large', SouthKrd. *ka<u>l</u>, ka<u>l</u>a* 'big', SulKrd. *ke<u>l</u>* 'strong, powerful, high', IrĀz. *kal* 'big' (REZĀZĀDE MALEK 1973 with further references), Gil. (Rāms.) *kal*- (only in compounds) 'big', Lo. *kala* 'big' (ADIB TUSI 1963–1964), Gz. *kal, käl* 'big, great; manly; eldest, chief of a human group'. In EIr., Yzγ. *qəl*-, probably never used as an independent lexical form, is also recorded in other compounds, such as *qəlxéx* 'large river', *qəlbawə́n* 'big hole in a mountain', *qəlbandáy* 'embankment', etc.

Prs. *kalān* 'big, massive, great' is well documented in the main dictionaries but is mostly used in Eastern Persian; see AfγPrs. *kalān* 'big, large', Xor.

kolū(n), Qāi. *kəlu*; Birǰ. *kalō*[*n*] 'old, aged (especially of sheep)', TrbHayd. *kulu(n), kolun* 'big'[157] and Taj. *kalon*.

Taj. *kalon* ~ (Iran) Prs. *bozorg* may be considered as one of the salient lexical shibboleths differentiating Tajik from Persian (LAZARD 1956: 180). In Boxārāi, *kalon* is the usual adjective for bigness in all possible extensions, and also includes reference to age. A different derivative from the same base is (Taj.) Vanǰ *kaluk* 'old' (ROZENFEL'D 1982).

The only MIr. antecedents we know are Man. Prth. *kalān* 'great, big'[158] and Khwar. *kl'*(*n*) 'big, great'. Cognates of, and sometimes direct loanwords from Prs. *kalān* are largely documented on the whole Iranian plateau. In many cases they have acquired the restricted, specialized meaning of 'senior; head of the village', and frequently occur in the comparative (cf. Prs. *kalāntar*). However, while *kalān* appears extraneous to the core lexicon of Standard Persian of Iran, its cognates are largely used in other WIr. languages, in particular Central dialects,[159] Southern Kurdish (Lakki, Kelhuri, Kermanšāhi[160]), Lori and Fārs dialects,[161] as well as in the languages spoken in North Iran (Caspian area).[162]

Different etymological proposals have been advanced for the *kalān*-group. According to ORANSKIJ (1970: 157–159), Prs. *kalān* / Taj. *kalon* has an EIr. origin; it should be considered as a loanword from some dialects having *l* < *t* (< OIr. **katā̆na-*; see also above p. 102). In view of Prth. *kalān*,

157 The relevant forms found in EIr. (Šγn. *kalōn*, Sgl. *kalān* 'big, large', Wx. *kalon* 'famous, great', Yzγ. *kalon* 'senior') are Prs. loanwords.

158 Note that there are two Man. Prth. (homographs or homophones?) words *q/kl'n*, the first meaning 'great', the second meaning 'pure' and being the equivalent of Sgd. *kr'n*, as first noticed by SIMS-WILLIAMS (1989: 329). According to SUNDERMANN (1994: 123 fn. 4) the meaning 'pure' makes better sense than 'great' in most passages in which Prth. *kl'n* occurs. The meaning 'great' may be admitted for only a few of them, while others remain ambiguous. Werner SUNDERMANN, whom I consulted on the matter, expounded his thinking in a letter sent to me on 19/11/2001; to him, for his usual kindness, go my heartfelt thanks.

159 Cf. Xuns. *kalun* 'big, out of size, plenty' (AŠRAF ALKETĀBI 1983: 445), Gz. *kälān* 'big, great', Krm. *kelān* 'big; large', Rāv. *kelūn* 'big', etc.

160 Krmnš. *kalen* 'big, great', Lak. *kalen* 'big (for people and things)', *kalén* 'big; senior; elder', (Tarhāni) *kaleyn* (HASURI 1964: 59). According to a chart in *Contrast of some Words in Kurdish dialects in Iran* [www.KurdDialectContrast.html, quoting *Awine* 25 (1375/1996), 81–83], Kelhuri/Lak. *ke̱ln* contrasts with SorKrd. and Awr. *gewre* 'big'.

161 Bxt. *kalon*, Lo. *kalo*, Dav. *kalun* 'leader; great'.

162 Cf. Gil. *klâ* 'big', Harz. *kala, kâlâ* 'big' and, eastwards, Dāmγāni *kalān* and Šahrudi *kelon* 'big' (ŠARIᶜATZĀDE 1992). See also *keleng* 'big, great' in the IrĀz. dialect of Lakestān, Šahrestān of Xoy, Western Azerbaijan (ADIB TUSI 1963–1964).

one might suppose that this word entered the Western plateau *via* Parthian, and penetrated into Tajik through a direct contact with an EIr. dialect spoken in the area of the historical Bactria. EILERS (1979: 681–682 s.v. *kal* and *kalān*) points to some kind of connection between *kal* and *kalān*, envisaging for *kal* a possible loan from Gr. κάρδακες 'mercenaries' (on which see SZEMERÉNYI 1971: 672, with literature, prospecting an Ir. origin for the Gr. word).

I would prefer considering Prs. *kalān* as an *ān*-derivative[163] from a base **kal*- 'big', whose modern outcomes have been mentioned above.

3.12. In Waxi, the thumb is named *lup yāŋgl* (IIFL-II, LORIMER 1958),[164] a lexicalized phrase containing the adjective *lup*, which means both 'big; adult; elder' and 'much'.

Wx. *lup* has unquestionable counterparts in a few EIr. languages: Išk. *lip*, Šγn., Roš., etc. *lap* 'much, many'; see also dial. Taj. *lum(b)* 'big; much, many' (ROZENFEL'D 1982). As possible cognates of Wx. *lup*, STEBLIN-KAMENSKIJ (1999 s.v.) also mentions Pšt. *loy, luy* 'big, large; adult; great, important; high (of voice)', as well as (Dardic) Bašgali *ola*', Aškun *aulú*, Kati *al* 'big', to which one could add Traieguma *úlláh* 'big' (LENTZ 1939: 197).

Without taking a definite stand on Pšt. *loy*,[165] I would connect Tāl. *yol* 'big; adult, senior' (*yol* in Anbarān Mahalle and Šânkāvar, *yul* in Jeid according to BAZIN 1981: 276) and Sang. *yâl(e)* 'big; tall' to the Dardo-Kafir forms mentioned above.

The presence of these items in languages spoken in North Iran could be attributed to a Turk. influence: cf. Turk. *ulu*, TurkĀz. *ulu* 'big'. The same could be true for Bašgali *ola*', Aškun *aulú*, Kati *al*, etc., for which in CDIAL 1211 an (unconvincing) protoform **āpula*- is reconstructed. Note that a connection between Turk. *ulu* and Pšt. *loy* had already been advanced in TOMASCHEK 1880: 816.

---

163 On the suffix *-ān* deriving adj. from adj. see HORN 1898–1901: 176.

164 As already noted by MORGENSTIERNE (IIFL-II), Wx. *hip i̯°* 'thumb' recorded in SKÖLD 1936: 141 should be explained as a misreading of a handwritten form *lup i̯°* in SKÖLD's original field notes.

165 See SKJÆRVØ 1989: 398 (< **dahăkah*-); NEVP 47 («A derivation < Av. *hu-δāta*- 'well-created, -built' is semantically unsatisfactory», with reference to NEVP 42). Both proposals have recently (and in my opinion rightly) been challanged by CHEUNG 2005: 129 («This word is possibly a regional borrowing, cf. Wa. *lap*, Sarik. *lɛwr* 'id.'»).

As a label for 'thumb' in Turkish-Mongol, one may quote OTurk. *uluγ ärṅäk*, lit. 'the big finger' (ERDAL 1981: 122) and probably Kalmyk *alae* quoted by POTT 1847: 297.

Is (South?) Krd. *âl* 'thumb' (EBRĀHIMPUR 1994b, s.v. *angošt*), recorded as *âl, yâḻ* 'middle finger' in HAŽĀR 1990 and EBRĀHIMPUR 1994a, to be put in connection with one of the lexical sets discussed in this paragraph? Should one analyse (South?) Krd. *âlxwâǰ* 'thumb' in EBRĀHIMPUR 1994b, s.v. *angošt* ('forefinger' in HAŽĀR 1990 and EBRĀHIMPUR 1994a), as a lexical compound containing *âl* and a reduced form of *xwâǰâ, xwâǰa* 'man of distinction, master', a term of respect that only a humanized, high-ranking finger might deserve?[166]

3.13. The thumb name in Koruni, a Krd. dialect spoken in Fārs, is *kelek-e qeyi*. The adjective *qeyi* 'big' (SALĀMI 2006: 189) is an Ar. lw. (cf. also Prs. *qavvi* 'strong, stout, robust') strongly integrated in the vocabularies of Kurdish, Lori, and surrounding areas. One may quote KurmKrd. *qewî* 'strong; very, very much', SouthKrd. *qavî* 'strong; powerful; sound and healthy; much, many', Krmnš. *qaüila* 'fat and huge' (*qä(y)ün* in *qä(y)ün-ü rân* 'Oberschenkel' CHRISTENSEN – BARR 1939: 353), Lo. *qevi* 'fat, robust, thick', Bxt. (ČLang) *qeyin* 'big, strong', Āvarz. *qey* 'big', Šušt. *gevend* 'fat and robust' (FĀZELI 2004), Vfs. *qævi* 'strong', Tāl. (Māsāl) *γavi* 'strong' (NAWATA 1982: 116), Siv. *kävīn* 'thick', recorded by ANDREAS (CHRISTENSEN – BARR 1939) but not confirmed by LECOQ's informants (1979: 200), etc.

3.14. Oss. *xīstær/xestær* means 'elder'; to it also belong Ydγ. *xušči*, Mnǰ. *xūšḱī, xūšḱəy, xuškī* 'greater, elder'. OIr. and MIr. antecedents (superlative forms) are Av. *hvōišta-* 'first; best', Khot. *hvāṣṭa-* 'best, chief, pre-eminent', Sgd. *xwyštk, γwyštk*, etc. 'teacher', (Man.) *xwyštr, xwštr* 'chief; superior'. As outcomes of old comparatives from the same base, we have Šγn. *xiđīr* (m.), *xadār* (f.) 'bigger, elder, grown up' (EVŠG), Haz. *γadār* 'much, many; large', AfγPrs. *xadal* 'big and disagreeable man'.

Oss. *xīstær æng₀ylʒ, ~ k'ūx*, Mnǰ. *xuški agūšḱa* and *xūšḱəgha*, Šγn. *xidār aŋgixt*, Roš. *xaïd iŋgaxt*, Šahdara *xada·r aŋgixt* (SKÖLD 1936: 186) 'thumb' are therefore figurative expressions, stressing on the social hierarchy (based on age or rank) characterizing humanized fingers.[167]

---

[166] An instance of a similar shortened form is Dav. *xoǰ* 'master, sir'.

[167] The thumb may depicted as the 'eldest (brother etc.)' in Modern IA as well; see CDIAL 5286 s.v. *jyēṣṭha-* 'first, chief', *jyēṣṭhá-* 'eldest; eldest brother'.

3.15. Prs. *angošt-e samin* 'thumb', recorded in traditional dictionaries but unknown to my Prs. informants, contains *samin* 'fat, full, plump', an Ar. loanword; cf. Ar. *samīn* 'fat, corpulent, plump; thick'.

3.16. Par. *ghaṇḍ* 'big; elder', occurring in Par. *ghaṇḍ γošt* (also *aŋgušt-e ghaṇḍ*) 'thumb', is a word of IA origin; cf. CDIAL 4424.

4. Though thumbs are thicker than other fingers, they are at the same time relatively short, or, we could say, of a quite low stature, if equated to human beings. This physical feature has been considered as conceptually salient and has favoured the creation of thumb designations in some languages in the world. In Gondi (a central Drav. language), for example, it is just this peculiarity to be emphasized: see *munḍā wiring* (*irinj*) 'thumb' (lit. 'the short finger') in DED^2 4938. In Lithuanian, the word for 'dwarf' (*nyštukas*) has been derived from the name of the thumb (*nykštis*). Note that the character known as *Poucet* in French (from Perrault's tale *Le Petit Poucet*; cf. also Engl. *Tom Thumb*, Germ. *Däumling*, It. *Pollicino* etc.) represents a perfect prototype of a dwarfish man.

Prs. *angošt-e kutāh* 'thumb', lit. 'the short finger', quoted in MOKRI 2005: 263, is the only instance I found in Iranian of this iconomastic pattern.

5. We have seen above (§ 3.11) a few *kal*-forms meaning 'big, great'. There are also *kal*-forms that mean (or *also* mean) 'male; strong':[168] male animals, such as he-goats, he-lambs or oxen, are often designated *kal*.[169] How the notions of MALENESS and PHYSICAL STRENGTH may be associated to the notion of BIGNESS is easily understandable: it is a fact of common human experience that males have bigger and stronger bodies than females. Here the question arises whether the *kal*-labels for 'thumb' mentioned in § 3.11 should be interpreted as "big/great fingers" or as "male fingers", as suggested by CHRISTENSEN – BARR (1939) for Kurd. (Garr.) *kelik e kal* and by EILERS (1979) for Gz. *kal*. It is not easy to take a stance. If it is true that the thumb finds in its physical dimension a natural motivation for its name, it is likewise true that in human imagery it is often equated to a living being,

---

[168] Cf. e.g. Gil. (Māč.) *kal* 'male', (Rāms.) *kal* 'male; big (in compounds)', etc.

[169] Cf. Prs. *kal* 'the male of any animal' with countless cognates in other languages. MAŠKUR (1978) compares Prs. *kal* with Hebrew *kar*, Akk. *kerru* 'he-lamb, ram'.

and recognized not only as the eldest of the group, but also as a member of the male category.

This associative conceptual relation also underlies Prs. *angošt-e nar, nar-angošti* (DEHX), which is in fact a lexical peculiarity of Eastern Persian:[170] cf. Taj. *narangušt* (KALBĀSI 1995 *nar-čilik*) and AfγPrs. *angošt-i nar* (ŠĀLČI 1991). In EIr., one finds Sgl. *naraŋgɜšt,* Mnǰ. *naraŋγušt,* Ydγ. *naraŋgušč,* Par. *narā̃ⁿ γošt,* Yγn. *narankŭšt* 'thumb'. Wx. *y̌əṣ̌-yaŋgl(ək)* (IIFL-II *γəṣ̌i-yāŋgəl*) 'thumb' similarly contains *y̌əṣ̌* 'male'.

It is possible that some of the EIr. *nar*-expressions for 'thumb' quoted above are due to a Taj. or AfγPrs. influence. However, Sogdian speakers could also have conceived the thumb as a "male finger", as proved by the Sgd. label *naršak* (<n(r)šk'>) 'thumb' (< 'little man'), recorded in a Sgd. list of body-parts (SUNDERMANN 2002: 144 and fn. 74).[171] To the thumb as a "male finger" also point some labels found in North Iran, namely Sang. *nar-angošt,* Lāsg. *nar-engošt,* Srx. *nōr-angošt,* Šahm. *nar-angošt.*

In fact, in a way specular to *kal*, for which one could envisage a BIG → MALE conceptual transfer, *nar* 'male' may acquire the additional sense of 'big'. This is suggested by MORGENSTIERNE for Ydγ.-Mnǰ. *nar-* («*nar* as a prefix indicates size or strength», IIFL-II, s.v. *narkafčī*) and by KIEFFER for Kab. *nar* («comme adj. ou en composition /*nar*/ peut signifier «grand, fort»», 1979–1980 s.v. *narãn*).[172] However, to consider the *nar*-fingers mentioned above as belonging to the "big finger" iconomastic type would be fully unjustified.

The "male-thumb" figurative expression is present in many languages in the world.[173] I limit myself to mention here Mongol *eregei chorogon* 'thumb' (cf. *ere* 'man; manly') and Kalmyk *irrekei* 'thumb' (cf. *irre, ere, aere* 'man'), quo-

---

170 Persian speakers from Tehran which I have asked for on several occasions have not recognized this expression as an acceptable name for thumb.

171 R. SCHMITT (p.c.) observes that Sgd. *naršak* cannot be analysed as *narš-ak* (as one could possibly be led to assume from SUNDERMANN's annotation «I.e. *naršak* 'little man', from Av. *narš* 'man' (Nom.) ? »), but only as *nar-°*, being Av. *narš* a gen. form. Though the morphological structure of the Sgd. word remains to be better defined, the actual connection of Sgd. *naršak* to the *nar*-finger names seems to me very probable.

172 Similarly, one might interpret Dašt. *narre* 'huge, bulky (of people and things)', Buš. *narre* 'ugly; coarse; bulky' ('(too) big' → 'graceless, ugly' is a predictable semantic shift in Iranian). See also Xuns. *nartevar* 'a kind of big hatchet', as compared to *tevar* 'hatchet'.

173 In the Turk. dialect spoken in Ruh-Ābād, a Southeastern dialect of Xorāsān Turkish, the thumb is said *hämuⁿ šast* (DOERFER – HESCHE 1993: 236), an idiom in which *šast* (loanword < Ir.) is modified by *hämuⁿ* 'male'.

ted by POTT 1847: 297, since here certainly belongs Haz. *erka* (Besut *ireka,* Daizangī *eratka*, DULLING 1973) 'thumb', one of the many Mongol/Kalmyk elements in Hazaragi. As far as IA is concerned, note Skt. *vr̥ṣo 'ṅgulinām* 'the chief among fingers, the thumb'; cf. Skt. *vŕ̥ṣan-* 'male, strong, etc.' in EWA II: 575f.

6. Since Prs. *nar* and cognates are neutral as to the nature of living beings referred to, the image evoked by the thumb names listed in the previous paragraph might be that of either a 'humanized' or an 'animalized' male finger. The animal world is surely the source domain for the conceptual association that has produced the "ram-finger" type denominations for thumb in Kurdish: cf. KurmKrd. *tilîya beranî, beranekê, beranek,*[174] SouthKrd. *barânê* (EBRĀHIMPUR 1994b *dipilâ barânê* s.v. *angošt*, SAFIZĀDE 2001 *barânkê, barânak*), all of them derivatives, or lexicalized phrases containing a derivative from Krd. *beran/barân*[175] 'ram'.

7. Attributing to fingers a kinship relationship represents a universal, having a worldwide, albeit discontinuous, distribution. In particular, the thumb is often equated to a parent: sometimes to an unspecified parent,[176] in few cases to a father, mostly to a mother.[177] The important role played by the thumb, as well as its strong constitution and its isolated position with respect to the other fingers, may account for this association, through which people ascribe to the thumb the role of a guide and guardian of the others.[178]

---

[174] Note the conflict between the conceptual category and the morphological gender; Krd. *beranek* is feminine, just as *tilya berenekê* is, since *tilî* 'finger' is a fem. word.

[175] For etymological references, see CHYET 2003 s.v.

[176] See e.g. Japanese *oyayubi* 'thumb' (lit. 'parent-finger').

[177] For more details, see BROWN – WITKOWSKI 1981: 601–602 (Table 4), where examples from different languages are listed. Further instances are *ne.kpe* (mother-hand) 'thumb' in Monzombo, a language from the Niger-Congo family (THOMAS 1981: 349); Malayam *ta<u>ll</u>a viral* 'thumb' (from *ta<u>ll</u>a* 'mother') and Parji *tal vanda* 'thumb' (from *tal* 'mother') in Dravidian (DED[2] 3136).

[178] Cultural expressions other than denomination processes may reveal the same human attitude towards their fingers, though the images evoked may vary. By way of illustration, consider the following Dezfuli riddle: *čiya čiya buniya dokuniya čâr bozenø: čupuniya*? (EMĀM 2000: 97) «What is this? There is a roof, there is a shop, four goats and one shepherd». The solution is: *dasø: kelekâ* ('the hand and the fingers') and may be explained in this way (ibid. fn. 1): the roof (*bun*, Prs. *bām*) represents each swelling at the bottom of the fingers; the shop (*dokun*, Prs. *dokkān*) represents the hollow in the palm of the hand; the shepherd (*čupun*, Prs. *čupān*) represents the thumb (which is obviously considered as a leader), while the four goats (*boz*) are the remaining fingers.

As derived from SBal. *māt*, WBal. *mās*, EBal. *māθ* 'mother', one may quote the following Bal. labels for thumb: *mātī* (*mātak* recorded from an Omani Bal. speaker), optionally followed by *lankuk* 'finger', widespread in SBal., with the exception of Karachi[179] and *māsī lankuk* or *māsīnk* (Panǰgūr). MORGENSTIERNE (1932a: 40) records *mātī*[180] *angul* from a Bal. speaker of Noške. For EBal., MAYER (1910 s.v. *thumb*) and HETU RAM (1898) provide *māθani murdānaγ* and *māθkī mordānaγ*[181] respectively. However, EBal. speakers I asked about, claimed to have never heard any of these expressions, or anything resembling them, so I do not know if and where they are (or were) actually used.

According to SAYAD HASHMI 2000, Bal. *mātī*, which basically means 'maternal', has the additional meaning of 'big, great, important, etc.'. The association of the notion of MOTHER with that of BEST REPRESENTATIVE of any category, perceived as the origin and the paradigm, is well known in the Middle East. However, though one may find a few Bal. instances of *māt*-compounds (such as *mātband* 'big embankment', *mātšāh* 'the main branch of a river' etc.), there is no evidence of any consistent usage of Bal. *māt* in the sense of 'big'. Therefore, there is no reason to interpret Bal. *mātī lankuk* as "the big finger" rather than "mother-finger".

In addition to the Bal. "mother-finger", we have at least another "parent-finger" in Iranian, in this case a "father-finger". It is found in the Fārs dialect of Kāzerun, where the thumb is named *bovaki*, a derivative from *bovo* 'father'.

8. If Prs. *šahin* is a phonetic variant of *šāhin* 'regal' (a derivative from *šāh* 'king'), the Prs. label *angošt-e šahin* 'thumb' would emphasize the importance attached to this finger. However, the scanty lexicographical documentation of this lexicalized phrase (see DEHX) make its presence in Persian at least dubious (a dialectal form?). To find a sure "regal" thumb one should look at Vfs. *šangoštœ, šahœngošte* (MOQDAM 1949), Āšt. *šā angošt*, Āmor. *šâšgonda* (*šā angošt* MOQDAM 1949) 'thumb', and dial. Taj. *šalik* (ROZENFEL'D 1982), which means 'thumb' in the area of Darvāz, where *lik* is the usual word for 'finger'.

---

179 The Karachi Bal. name of the thumb is *gaḍḍī* (see below p. 139).

180 Actually *matī* in MORGENSTIERNE (ibid.); this form could be explained as a misprint, a mishearing or a contextual phonetic variant of *mātī* produced by the speaker.

181 MORGENSTIERNE (1932a: 40) did not recognize in these words the base *māθ* 'mother' and hinted (with his annotation «$\theta = z$?») at possible variants of *mazan* 'big'. Analogously, I think that MORGENSTIERNE did not recognize the connection of *matī angul* (recte *mātī*; see fn. 180 above) with *māt* 'mother'.

Further instances of a "regal finger" (or better a "very important finger")[182] will be met with in the following chapters: the thumb shares this iconomastic pattern with both the fore- and the middle finger.

9. Taj. *sarangušt*[183] 'thumb' is equivalent to Turk. *başparmak* 'thumb' and lit. means 'the finger at the head'. From a Panǰgūri Bal. speaker I have recorded *lankuke sarag* 'thumb', but the syntactic structure of this expression, different from the one expected in Bal., with the dependence construction moving towards left, points to an external influence (Persian or Balochi of Ir. Sarāwān?).

However, Taj. *sarangušt*, which apparently depicts the thumb as a leader, could also be explained resorting to another motivation: it could point to the position of the thumb in comparison with the other fingers, describing it as the finger coming first ('at the head') in the topography of the hand.

10. Killing lice by swatting them seems to have been a task for which the thumb has proved to be particularly functional.[184] It is one of the functions fulfilled by this finger that has beaten the human imagination, and influenced naming processes in many languages.

In Iranian, a few thumb names diffused in the South/Central Kurdish area provide evidence for this argument. They are Sor. *espêkuje* (pop.) (HAKIM 1996), *qamkî espêkuže* (KURDOEV – JUSUPOVA 1983), SouthKrd. *espê kuže* (*sipîa kuža* EBRĀHIMPUR 1994a), Krmnš. *šepeš košak*. They have parallels in Central Iran and in South-Eastern Iran; compare ZorYzd. *šepeš košōg*, Xur. *spež kož* (ŠĀYEGĀN 2006: 171), Rod. *šoškošak*. All these expressions share iconym, lexical structure and etymology: they are lexical compounds with agentive forms of the verb 'to kill' governing the word for 'louse' as their object ('(the one) who kills lice'). Min. *marge šošon,* NBšk. (Sardašt) *marge rešon*, SBšk. (Garu) *marge xešan* (G. BARBERA p.c.) 'thumb' rest on the same motivational pattern. In these dialects, however, through a metonymi-

182 Prs. *šāh, šah* 'king', as well as its several cognates in many Ir. languages, is commonly used to form nominal compounds referring to high-level members inside a category. Instances are Prs. *rāh* 'road' vs. *šāhrāh* 'main road, highway', *tut* 'berry' vs. *šāhtut* 'black mulberry', etc.

183 Not to be confused with Taj. *sarangušt* 'tip of the finger', i.e. the 'head (upper part) of the finger'.

184 In Gilaki, this practice was called *čungul*. For this operation (*čungul zēn*), people generally used to help each other, and especially women used not to go to sleep before having performed it (BOŠRĀ 2002: 213).

cal association (intra-domain mapping), the thumb is directly equated to the effect of its action, i.e. death (*marg*); it is conceived as 'the death of lice'.[185]

In favour of the fact that many people in the world (and not only the Kurds, or the Zoroastrians of Yazd or the inhabitants of some SE Iranian areas) have found it expedient when necessary to get rid of lice using their own thumbs, also speak the corresponding Mediterranian figurative expressions for 'thumb' pointed out by SERRA (1971–1973: 445–446), viz. *accíra prúkkju* or *skázza prúkkju* (lit. 'the killer [or the swatter] of lice') in a few dialects of Basilicata (Italy); *igémz* (lit. '[the one which] swats') in the Berber variety spoken in Zuwāra (Libya) and *gaṭṭā el-gúmla* ('[the one which] swats the lice') in the Ar. dialect spoken in Tripoli. Similar denominations are found in Northern Italy (Alta Valtellina), as *mizaciöc'* (Alboseggia), *mazaplögl* (Livigno), *mazza piöcc* (Brianza), etc. (BRACCHI 2009: 286). One may also produce several instances of finger-rhymes for children where the thumb is introduced in its capacity as lice-killer (Arabic: CHEBEL 1999: 88–89; Low German: POTT 1847: 293, also VEENKER 1981: 375).

The "lice-killer" thumb is generally felt as a popular designation; it is therefore doomed to be cancelled from the lexicon of each language in its normalization phases.

11. Long time before the uniqueness of fingerprints was recognized, and long before the signature was currently used to validate documents, fingers and nails[186] had an important function in the bureaucratic procedures. They were used as individual seals of acts in many cultural environments, though according to different practices. As demonstrated by KUMAMOTO (1987b), Khotanese people used the Chinese and Tibetan "finger-seal" method (Chin. *huazhi*), i.e. drawing lines symbolizing the shape and length of fingers at the end of documents, while there is no Khot. evidence of an alternative usage of the Chinese method (*zhiyin*) that consisted of making a fingerprint (probably with the thumb) over the personal name. Consequently, Khot. *haṃguṣṭa* (other spelling *hagauṣṭa*) 'finger', occurring at the end of many Khot. documents along with personal names, has to be interpreted as 'finger-seal', and not 'finger-mark'. However, the practice of making fingerprints as substitutes for sig-

[185] Note that dialects of that area have different words for 'louse'; in some it is *šoš* (cf. Prs. *šepeš* and cognates 'id.'), in others it is *reš* (cf. Prs. *rešk* and cognates 'nit'); in the SBšk. dialect of Garu it is *xešk* (G. BARBERA p.c.).

[186] For the usage of nails to validate documents in Mesopotamia, see EBELING 1957; in Bactria, see SIMS-WILLIAMS 2000: 112, 113 doc. U27, etc.

natures by illitterates should have been widespread on the Ir. plateau. It has survived in culturally peripheral areas, as is proved by an episode described by BALSAN in the account of his travel in Bašākerd in late 1967 («Ali Nushirwani accepta, à condition que l'accord fût transcript sur un bout de papier signé par moi et par le Sayed Reza [...] Puis il apposa son pouce», 1969: 264). Evidence is also provided by the Siv. idiom *gos vin deyan* 'signer avec le pouce enduit d'encre' (LECOQ 1979). KurmKrd. *tilya navnîşanê* 'thumb' (AMÎRXAN 1992), containing *navnîşan* 'sign, token, marking', could be explained resorting to the 'signing' function performed by the finger.

12. The botanical world has probably served as the domain source for metaphorical associations that produced a couple of labels recorded in South Kurdish. These are *nâl* (EBRĀHIMPUR 1994b s.v. *angošt*) and (Mahâb.) *tilyâ gizrê* (AWRANG 1969); cf. *nâl* 'thin string of reed' and *gizre* 'thorn, straw'.

13. As all the other fingers, the thumb may be designated with terms whose primary meaning is (or originally was) 'finger' (semantic change), or which derive from words for 'finger'.[187] In Iranian, one finds Sed. *uŋguss* and Wan. *nguṭā* (also 'fore- and middle finger'),[188] both belonging to the *angošt*-type group (see above, pp. 56 ff.).[189] Similarly, Sor./SulKrd. *qamk* 'thumb' (HAKIM – GAUTHIER 1993, s.v. *pouce*) is originally one of the (South/Central) Krd. words for 'finger' (see above p. 84), while Bast. *angošt bačo,* Farām. *boča, bača* 'thumb' could be connected with Phl. *bačag* for which see above p. 86.

Khot. *āṣṭī, āṃṣṭī* 'thumb' probably falls into the same iconomastic typology. It derives from **anguštiya-* 'connected with fingers' (BAILEY 1979) or **anguštika-* (DEGENER 1989), with a compensatory lengthening.

Khot. *āṣṭī* induces the following digression on an Av. word that sounds similar to the Khot. form, without being etymologically related.

Y. 9.11 and *Yt.* 19.40, two parallel passages with minor differences, recall the killing of the mythical hero Kərəsaspa by Aži Sruuara, the poisonous, horse-devouring, men-devouring yellow serpent, on which yellow, *ārštyō-barəzan-* poison grows. Taking into account «Skt. *muchtyaguchttha*, lit. 'le pouce du poing'», with which Neryosangh translates Av. *ārštyō-barəzan-*, BURNOUF (1845: 270–271), suggested interpreting *ārštyō-* as 'pouce'. Many

187 A few examples in Slavonic languages are provided in VEENKER 1981: 364.

188 «Borr. from Lhd. *aŋgūṭhā*, but influenced by *n^{ə}gut* 'finger'» (MORGENSTIERNE 1930: 168).

189 For IA parallels see Skt. *aṅguṣṭhá-* and cognates in CDIAL 137.

subsequent translations of these Av. passages have been influenced by BURNOUF's understanding. According to MILLS (1887: 234), from the body of the terrifying snake, «as thick as thumbs are, greenish poison flowed aside» (*Y.* 9.11). Similarly, DARMESTETER (1883: 295) translated «yellow poison flowed of a thumb's breadth» the parallel passage *Yt.* 19.40. A new interpretation of *ārštyō-barəzan-* ('von Klafterhöhe') and consequently of *Y.* 9.11 («auf dem das Gift klafterhoch floss») is advanced by BARTHOLOMAE (1904), who explains *ārštyō-* as derived from **ārštya-* 'Höhe, Lange eines Speers', «Ableit. aus» *arštya-* 'Speer, Lanze'.

BARTHOLOMAE's suggestion has generally been accepted by Western scholars (see lastly HINTZE 1994: 212 and HUMBACH – ICHAPORIA 1998: 116–117), but never fully accepted in Zoroastrian circles; compare KANGA 1909 (s.v. *thumb*) and BAHRĀMI 1990, where Av. *ārštya-* is still recorded as 'thumb'.

Notwithstanding the clear, general sense, the proper understanding of the relevant passages has been a question ever since. Even the Pahlavi translator of *Y.* 9.11 should not have grasped too much of the original Avestan text, at least judging from *asp-bālāy*, i.e. 'to the height of a horse'[190] which translates Av. *ārštyō-barəzan-*, not to mention the long rambling gloss (quoted in HUMBACH – ICHAPORIA 1998: 117) that he felt the need to add in order to justify his translation. And certainly Neryosangh had troubles in translating into Sanskrit, as well. However, which reasoning led him to produce the odd compound «*muchtyaguchttha*» is really very difficult to understand. It is plausible that since the topic was about a dimensional value, Neryosangh thought to introduce an element commonly used as a measure of length, and the thumb meets the case perfectly. Even the context (poison growing over a surface) could have favoured the recourse to a small measure, like a finger, rather than a big one, like a spear or a similar object. May Neryosangh have been influenced by the assonance with some cognate(s) of Khot. *āṣṭī* 'thumb', also used as a measure of length,[191] or Av. *ašti-* 'four fingers' breath, palm'?

14. Ar. *ibhām* 'thumb, big toe' has found its way in Persian and has become a (very) formal alternative to *šast*; cf. Prs. (*angošt-e*) *ebhām* 'thumb,

---

190 Note that the Phl. translator resorted to a conventional expression which also occurs elsewhere in Phl. texts and is used to emphasize the big dimension of a specific element; cf. *WZ* 16.3.

191 Cf. *āṣṭye āṣṭye mase gvīhä: rruṃ jsa gūmalyāñä* "to size of a thumb each with butter to be smeared on" (*Siddhasāra* 122rl; quoted in BAILEY 1979 s.v. *āṣṭī*).

great toe', Taj. *angušt-i ibhom*. At first sight, this Ar. label could seem to represent the thumb as "the finger of the ambiguity"; cf. Ar. *ibhām* 'obscurity, ambiguity', also found in Persian as a loanword (*ebhām*). This should have been, at least according to my knowledge, a figurative expression with no check from any other (Iranian and non-Iranian) languages. In fact, Ar. *ibhām* 'thumb' and *ibhām* 'ambiguity' are merely homonyms; the former belongs (with «-*m* < *-*n* by assimilation to *b*-») to the same root as Akk. *ubānu, upānu* 'finger, toe' and the related Semitic words collected in MILITAREV – KOGAN 2000: no. 34, already quoted above p. 90.

15. In Balochi, three different names for thumb represent isoglosses with a clear-cut areal distribution: *šast* characterizes WBalochi, *mātī* characterizes SBalochi, while the most usual thumb name in EBalochi, practically unknown in other Bal. varieties, is *deb/ḍeb*.[192] This latter word, which has not been recorded with any other meanings in Bal. dictionaries and glossaries, seems at first sight to have an Indian origin, but I have found no Indian language, whether contiguous or not with the Bal. area, in which the name of the thumb somehow resembles *ḍeb/deb*. Is there any connection with Krd. *tipil/dipil* 'finger' seen above pp. 90 f.? I also have no suggestion as regards the etymology and iconym of one of the Pšt. labels for 'thumb', viz. *báṭa* (*gúta*), and one of the thumb names recorded in Fārs, viz. Dāreng. *penǰe-y šāδi* and Nud. *penǰe-y šad*.

Oss. *muč'a* 'thumb', which was given to me by speakers from different Ossetic areas, is not commented in IESOJ. Caucasian origin?

[192] Also *dep, dīp/díp*, according to DAMES 1891, MAYER 1910 and GILBERTSON 1925.

CHAPTER FOUR: THE FOREFINGER

1. The forefinger is commonly used by people all over the world to indicate something by pointing to it. In naming this finger, laying emphasis upon the pointing function has proved to be one of the most predictable iconomastic patterns.[193]

Late Skt. *deśinī-, pradeśinī-* 'forefinger' (EWA III: 269) may be referred to the verb *diśáti* 'points out' (CDIAL 6340, EWA I: 744–746), generally connected to IE **deik̂-* 'to show, point' (IEW 188–189), to which Lat. *digitus*[194] (> It. *dito*) 'finger', Lat. *index* (> It. *indice*) 'index finger', etc. also belong. Skt. *diṣṭi-* 'a measure of length' (CDIAL 6343; EWA I: 745) is connected to the same verb as Skt. *deśinī-*, etc. An Ir. counterpart of Skt. *diṣṭi-* is Av. *dišti-* 'ein Längemass' (BARTHOLOMAE 1904), which, according to *FrO* (XXVIIa), is equivalent to ten fingers.[195] In the scale of values, a *dišti-* is shorter than a *vītasti-* and longer than an *uzašti-*, the last two being equivalent to twelve and eight fingers respectively (BARTHOLOMAE 1904; *FrO* ibid.). Modern Ir. and IA cognates of Av. *dišti-*[196] and *vītasti-*[197] are all recorded with the meaning 'span', i.e. the distance between (outstretched) thumb and (outstretched) little finger. However, if Av. *vītasti-* seems to be what is called a 'large span', Av. *dišti-* could be a 'small span', i.e., the distance between (outstretched) thumb and (outstretched) forefinger, equivalent to Prs. *fetr* (< Ar.).[198]

All things considered, I suggest taking Av. *dišti-* as a name of, or as a form somehow related to an unattested name of the forefinger, etymological-

193 Forefinger names based on this motivation are numberless; for a few instances see VEENKER 1981: 368–369.

194 A collection of different etymologies for Lat. *digitus* is in ANDRÉ 1991: 99; for a new proposal on the formation of this word (nominalization from adverb) see SILVESTRI 2000: 123 fn. 20.

195 Cf. also Phl. *dišt* in *FrO* (ibid.) and in the *Supplementary Texts to the Šāyest nē-šāyest*, XVI.4 (KOTWAL 1969).

196 Cf. Oss. *dīsny* (IESOJ) and CDIAL 6343.

197 A collection of cognate forms is in IESOJ s.v. *wydīsn(y)*. See also ELFENBEIN 1992: 250–251.

198 According to KLINGENSCHMITT (1968: 239), Av. *dišti-* «bezeichnet die beiden Handbreiten und gehört wohl zur Wz. diś 'zeichen'».

ly connected with *daēs-* 'to show, point'.[199] Skt. *prādeśinī-* 'a span long; the forefinger', *prādeśá-* 'the span of the thumb and forefinger, etc.', *pradeśa-* 'pointing out, showing; a short span (measured from the tip of the thumb to that of the forefinger), etc.', as compared with *deśinī-* and *pradeśinī-* quoted above, could support such an assumption. Consider also Gr. λιχάς 'the space between the forefinger and thumb, the lesser span', hardly to separate from λιχανός 'forefinger' (see also CHANTRAINE 1980: 629).

Leaving aside Av. *dišti-*, whose etymology and primary meaning still require a deeper investigation, we may quote some Ir. expressions for 'forefinger' describing it as the "pointing finger" or the "sign finger". These are Prs. *angošt-e nešān*[200] (*nešān* 'sign'), Taj. *čilik-i-nišonte* ('the finger giving signs', KALBĀSI 1995), with their Krd. and Fārs dialect counterparts, e.g. KurmKrd. *t'ilîya nîşanê/nîşandekê/nîşankirinê* (RIZGAR 1993 *t'ilîya nîşandanê*), SouthKrd. *kilk nîšân* (SAFIZĀDE 2001), Dav. *pinǰe-y nušuna* (SALĀMI 2004), Knd. *penǰe-y nešuna,* Rič. *penǰe-y nošuna*, all of them meaning 'forefinger'.

Prs. *ešāre/ešārat* / Taj. *išorat* 'pointing with fingers; sign' occurs in Prs. *angošt-e ešāre/ešārat* / Taj. *angušt-i išorat* 'forefinger'. It is an early Ar. lw. from the root ŠWR.[201] Here also belongs Prs. *mošire, moširat* 'forefinger' (STEINGASS 1963). In Fārs, one finds Kor. *kelek-e ešâra*, Pāp. *penǰe-y ešâra* 'id.'.

Ar. *išāra* also entered the Khwar. lexicon; cf. *'š'rt* 'sign, wink'. The adjectival derivative *'š'rt-mync* occurs in the expression *y' 'š'rt-mync 'kwnd*, the Khwar. name of the forefinger.

The "pointing finger" type is not commonly used in Balochi, but does not have dialect restrictions; I have recorded EBal. (Mari) *išāraya murdānaγ*, as well as *išāra* and *nišāne lankuk*, these two latters from Ir. Bal. speakers.

In Ossetic, the forefinger is called *amonæn ængwylʒ*. Oss. *amonæn* derives from the verb *amonyn : amynd* 'to show, to advice'.

A "making signals" finger is also the image evoked by Prs. *angošt-e γammāz*, with *γammāz* 'ogling; shaking', from the Ar. root ΓMZ; cf. Ar. *g͟hamaza* 'to make a sign, to signal'.

---

199 See also Av. *dišti-* 'that which points out; index; a measure of half a span about five inches' in BAHRĀMI 1990 (with the somehow odd labels "*adabi*" / "Lit.").

200 A few Tehrāni speakers which I asked about, claimed that *angošt-e nešān,* differently from *angošt-e ešāre* and *angošt-e sabbābe*, is not a current forefinger name in Modern Persian, though it is well understood.

201 Cf. Ar. (II) *šawwara* 'to make a sign, to point out', (IV) *ašāra* 'to make a sign', etc.

While using fingers in order to send messages, human beings observe a gestural code shared by the members of the community to which they belong. Some of the codified signs, however, have proved to be common to different cultures. For instance, to draw somebody to oneself making signals with the forefinger is a very common practice. Surely, Sogdians used to do it as well, and they left trace of this practice in their lexicon. Sgd. *niwēδēne-angušt*, i.e. 'the inviting finger' (cf. *nw'yδ-* 'to invite; to inform') is the Sgd. forefinger name. It occurs in the Buddhist text P 14, 25 (BENVENISTE 1940).

In the communicative practice, the proxemic code interacts with the speech code. Taj. *angušt-i xitob* 'forefinger', lit. 'the finger of the approach', stresses upon the use of the forefinger in conversation; by moving it, the speaker intends to draw the addressee's attention.

2. Wagging or holding up one's forefinger may be a deprecatory gesture, with which one expresses disapproval, reproach and even contempt. The forefinger may be used in order to frighten or to insult, and this fact explains the labels reviewed in what follows.

Prs. (*angošt-e*) *sabbābe*,[202] Taj. (*angušt-i*) *sabboba* and Prs. *sebbat* (DEHX) are Ar. loanwords; cf. Ar. *sabbāba* 'index finger' (from *sabba* 'to insult, abuse'). Here also belongs Gz. *engolī-šäbbābe* 'forefinger'. Prs. *angošt-e došnām* and *došnām-dehande* contain *došnām* 'curse, execration'. The same human disposition towards this finger accounts for one of the late Skt. names of the forefinger, *tarjanī-* (cf. EWA III: 238, s.v. TARJ 'drohen, schelten').

Bal. *šābāš*, as well as Prs. *šādbāš, šābāš* and several Ir. cognates, is commonly used as an exclamation of approval ('bravo! well-done, congratulations'). Apparently, EBal. *šābāš murdānaγ*, provided to me by a Bugti speaker (but unknown to Bal. speakers from other areas), would point to the usage of this finger to express the feeling of liking and admiration for someone or something.[203] However, by means of contrast, an associative principle based in many cases on irony (as a rhetoric figure), Bal. *šābāš* may also become a mark of disproval; *šābāš kanag* has acquired the meaning of 'to curse, scold' (= *laᶜnat kanag*). Documentation (at least for the Raxšāni dialect) is given by Hans STRASSER in the *šābāš* cards included among the ca.

[202] Belonging to the literary language; cf. MOINFAR 1981: 230. G. BARBERA has recorded *sabâba* 'forefinger' in Mināb; this term was however perceived as a Prs. word by Min. speakers.

[203] This was also the interpretation proposed in FILIPPONE 2000–2003: 65.

40,000 of his planned Bal. dictionary (now kept in the Archive of the Austrian Academy of Sciences – *Nachlass Strasser*).[204]

The forefinger may also be used in order to show protection and mercy towards other people and this motivates Prs. *angošt-e zenhār* (or *zinhār*) and *angošt-e amān*, with *zenhār, zinhār* 'quarter, mercy, protection' and *amān* 'safety, quarter, peace'. Note, however, that Taj. *angušt-i zinhor* is recorded as one of the names of the ring finger.

The forefinger is the finger with which one may communicate to have doubts about something, to be somehow perplexed; hence, in Persian it is also called *angošt-e šak* (DEHX), lit. 'the finger of the doubt'. It may be used when cautioning someone against doing something, in giving advice; it is the finger most concerned with intellectual activities and knowledge; therefore, it may be referred to as *andām-e dānā* (DEHX, lit. 'the wise limb')[205] in Persian.

3. The forefinger is universally associated to the cultural domain of RELIGIOUSNESS: for this reason all over the world it may be referred to as 'the finger of the prayer' or similar expressions.[206]

Muslims hold up their forefingers during the declaration of faith, the *šahāda* ('witnessing'). It follows that the forefinger is the 'finger performing the *šahāda*', as evidenced by *aš-šāhid*, the Ar. label for 'forefinger', which has strongly influenced the forefinger denominations in many Muslim communities.

In Iranian, one may quote the following: Prs. *angošt-e šehādat,*[207] AfγPrs. *angɔšt-e šahādat* (BAU 2003), Taj. *angušt-i šahodat,* Lo. *kalak-e šāhed* (UNVALA 1958: 14), SorKrd. *qamkî šehade* (KURDOEV – JUSUPOVA 1983), SouthKrd. *šâda*; *šâda niwêž* (with *niwêž* 'prayer'), *angûs šâdat*, *dipilâ šâhidî* (EBRĀHIMPUR 1994b s.v. *angošt*), (Krmnš.) *angušt-e šādat,* (Garr.) *kelik e šâhat*, Lak. *šâhed*, Gor. (Gahw.) *kilik-i šāyid*, Zā. *gištā šādi*, Tāl. (Rep. of Azerbaijan) *šəadətə angištə* (PIREJKO 1976), (Kargānrudi) *šahodata angəšta* (D. GUIZZO p.c.), Šahm. *šahādat*, Kāz. *penǰe-y šâdat*, Gavk. *penǰēy šādat*, Dahl. *penǰe-y šâhâδat*, Mās., Dāreng., Dorun., Nud., Birov., Dādenǰ., Dusir., Mosq. *penǰe-y šâδat*, Kal. (Lor) *penǰe-y šaδat*, Dežg. *penǰe-y šâhâδe*, Abd., Somγ., Ban., Gorgn. *penǰe-y šâhâdat*, Baliā. *penǰe-y šahâdat,* Hay. *penǰe-y*

204 A preliminary report on Dr. STRASSER's *Nachlass* is available in ROSSI 2004–2006: 68–69.

205 Or 'the limb of the wise man'?

206 For a few instances, see VEENKER 1981: 369. The close link between the forefinger and the divine explains the concern expressed by this finger in the children-rhyme (a) quoted above, p. 49.

207 Tehrāni speakers perceive this Prs. term as a religious, legal term (REZĀI BĀΓBIDI p.c.).

šahāδe, Kal. (Tāǰ.) *penǰar-e šâdat*, Dašt. *pinǰe-y šâ:dat*, Bast. *angošt šahāda* 'forefinger'.

In Balochi, I have recorded *šahādate lankuk* (Makrān), *šahādate hor* (Noške), and *šahādat murdānaγ* (Mari); all of them, however, are formal terms, not used in everyday language. Koroši has *šahāδatey penǰa*.

QALANDAR MOMAND – SEHRAYI 1994 record Pšt. *šahādát gwə́ta* as a gloss to *šinγáṭa* 'forefinger'; Par. *aŋgušt-e šaådat* is clearly a Prs. loanword.

In AWRANG 1969: 294, Krd. (*tilîya*) *dalastokî* is glossed by Prs. *angošt-e gavāhi*; a phrase where *gavāhi* 'witness' replaces *šehādat* 'id.'.

With the forefinger, the worshipper gives witness of his own faith, but also appeals to God and eulogizes His name, as illustrated by Prs. *angošt-e allāhxān*, or *xodāxān, xodāvān* (DEHX) 'forefinger', with the present stem of the verb *xāndan* 'to call, etc.' as the second part of the compound,[208] and Prs. *mosabbehat*, a lw. from Ar. *musabbiḥa* 'forefinger', morphologically related to *sabbaḥa* 'to praise, glorify'.

Is it to God that one gives thanks with the forefinger, also called *angošt-e šokr* ('the finger of thanks'), as recorded by the traditional Persian dictionaries (DEHX)?

4. All the pious activities mentioned in the above paragraph pertain to the spiritual life and to the human relationship with the divine. However, other, more prosaic and earthly activities also play an important role in life, and it does not pay to be too finicky and disregard them. Wisely, human people have never done it and have taken them into consideration in denomination processes.

Eating is one of the most important human activities, being a prerequisite to life. The relevance of the forefinger in the act of eating, and especially in eating with the hands, is undeniable. However, nutrition (to which a sacral aspect may also be attributed) is only a part of the FOOD EATING conceptual domain, which also includes references to human attitudes towards food as pleasures dispenser (relish, greed, gluttony, avidity, etc.). This aspect is emphasized by the names of the forefinger depicting it as a "plate-licker" or something like that, which people from quite different cultures have created. The wide spreading of this figurative expression is surprising,[209] and even

---

[208] Prs. *angošt-e xodāxān* occurs in the *Kāmel at-Taᶜbīr*; cf. MOKRI 2005: 264. These idioms, however, are never used in everyday language.

[209] Cf. Gr. λιχανός 'forefinger' (lit. 'the licker' «from its use in licking up»); Lat. (< Gr.) *lichanos* (ANDRÉ 1991: 102). POTT provides a few examples in Slavonic (1847: 292) and Mongol (1847: 297; *dologhobor chorogon* 'forefinger', prob. from *dologhocho* 'to lick').

when not stabilized as the finger's "normal" name, it is used all the same in folk songs and folklore throughout the world.[210] Iranian provides many examples of this popular association.

Taj. *kosales* 'flatterer' (cf. Prs. *kāselis* 'flatterer; beggar, low fellow') is used (in local varieties?) with the meaning of 'forefinger' (recorded in STEBLIN-KAMENSKIJ 1999: 189). In Central Iran, we find Gz. *kāselis*, Xur. *tāvålēs*, *tāvåbelēs* (*tāvā leys* FARAHVAŠI 1976: 2), ZorYzd. *kōsa-līsōg* 'forefinger', lexicalized phrases containing the present stem with agentive function or the agentive form (Yzd. *līsōg*) of the verb 'to lick' (connected to Prs. *lisidan*), which governs a word for 'bowl' (Prs. *kāse*) or 'pot' (Xur. *tāvā*) as its object. Similarly, the forefinger is named *kāsag-līsok*, *āsag-līsok* (with loss of the initial velar), *kāsa-layso* in WBal. (Noške, Xārān), lexical compounds from *kāsa(g)* 'plate, bowl' and *līsag* 'to lick'. Bal. (Kalāt) *kāsa-čaṭ* simply differs from the just mentioned idioms in that it contains the present stem of *čaṭṭag* 'to lick'. In my fieldwork in Balochistan, I noticed that the "bowl-licker" forefinger was used (or accepted) only by WBal. speakers, and even not by all of them.[211] However, this figurative expression is found in dictionaries and glossaries of other Bal. varieties as well: cf. *kāsag čatūk* (COLLETT 1983; basically Makrāni), *kāsagč^{h}at* (HETU RAM 1898; MAYER 1910 s.v. *finger*; EBal.). Br. *kāsalēs* 'forefinger' may be a Bal. lw. or derive from another Ir. source (ROSSI 1979: H628).

The present stem of *lapiden* 'to lick' is involved in the formation of Min. *kāsalap* 'forefinger' (G. BARBERA p.c.), which has parallels in Baškardi; cf.

SERRA (1971–1973: 445–446) quotes *lekká pjatt* ('plate licker') in a dialect of Basilicata (Southern Italy), *alḥas* ('(who) licks') in the Zuwāra Berber variety (Libya), *haṣṣal el-gáṣ^{c}a* ('(who) takes from the plate') in Tripolitan Arabic (see also the finger-rhymes quoted in CHEBEL 1999: 88–89). In Celtic, we find Breton *biz liper* ('the licker finger') and Cornic *lykka soresyow* ('the lick dregs') (FLEURIOT 1981: 136). See also *lic(h)iaflór* (lit. 'cream-licker') in the dialect of Livigno and other dialects of Alta Valtellina, in Northern Italy (BRACCHI 2009: 286). Skt. has *annâdí-tamā-* 'forefinger', lit. 'eating the most' (ŚBr.).

210 Some Ir. Bal. speakers from Sarāwān reported to me a children rhyme where each line is devoted to a finger, starting from the thumb (see below, p. 140); in it, the forefinger happens to be named *kāsag-līsok*. They told me that this forefinger name is used only in this rhyme and only by children. Likewise, in a nursery rhyme in Low German (POTT 1847: 293; also VEENKER 1981: 375), very similar to the Bal. one, the forefinger is styled "potlicker".

211 The data I have collected are somehow conflicting; a Bal. speaker from Xārān, for example, gave it to me as unusual; another one, native to the same town, maintained that he currently used it as the name of the forefinger.

NBšk. (Sardašt) *kosalap*, SBašk. (Angoran) *kosa lappošt*, (Garu) *kāsalap* (G. BARBERA p.c.).

The forefinger is also depicted as a "licker" in Kurdish, both in Northern and Southern dialects; compare Kurm. *tilîya fira̱xalîsk̲ê* (RIZGAR 1993), i.e. 'the one who licks pots and pans' (cf. *alast̲in* 'to lick' and *firaq* 'pots and pans; the dishes') and *tilîya dalastokî* (SAFIZĀDE 2001) 'forefinger', from *dalastin* 'to lick'. See also SorKrd. *(qamkî) došawmiže* (KURDOEV – JUSUPOVA 1983), SouthKrd. *(qâmkî) došâwmiža* (HAŽĀR 1990), *angustî došāw miža* (SAFIZĀDE 2001), a compound of *došaw* 'syrup of grapes' and *miž-*, from *mižīn* 'to suck'. The syrup of grapes is also evoked in one of the Gilaki forefinger names, *dušo-xori-angušt*, (Māč.) *dušâb xor angüšt*. In Abiānei, one finds *angöšta halīmxare* 'forefinger', i.e. the 'finger eating the *halim*'.

The "licker-finger" iconomastic type is also attested in EIr.; cf. Roš. *δakēc*, Šγn. *δakīǰak angix̌t* and Baǰ. *δakiǰak ingax̌t* 'forefinger', all of them lit. meaning 'the licker (finger)' (cf. *δak- : δikt* 'to lick'). Some problems arise in interpreting Wx. *yi:tokaiaŋgl* 'forefinger', quoted by LORIMER 1958. However, LORIMER's suggestion,[212] i.e. a tentative connection between *yi:tok* and the verb *yaw- : yit-* 'to eat', could have a leg to stand on, being supported by what has been said above.

The forefinger names listed above reflect a sort of blame towards this finger. They do not portray it as a just eating finger, but rather as a greedy finger, eating piggishly. The meaning 'flatterer', with its negative implications, of Prs. *kāselis* or KurmKrd. *firaqalês* (RIZGAR 1993) reinforces this assumption. And that this finger, because of its avidity, is not immune from censure is also proved by the name used by the Waxi speakers, *y̌udyangl(ək)* ('the thief (*y̌ud*) finger'). In Old Turkish as well, the forefinger (*suq ärṅäk*) is 'the finger of the avidity'; the same happens in Kazakh, Kirghiz, Turkmen and other modern Turkish languages. Kāšğarī (11th c. Turkish lexicographer) explains the Turkish label pointing out the fact that the forefinger is the finger moving first when is time to take food (ERDAL 1981: 123).

5. The EATING FOOD domain could probably also explain Western Pšt. *miswā́k gúta* 'forefinger' (RAVERTY 1860), *moswā́ka gwə́ta* (QALANDAR MOMAND – SEHRAYI 1994), being *miswā́k, moswā́k* a stick from a particular

212 «Can yi:tok represent an alternative form to yi·tn 'to eat' ?» (LORIMER 1958, not numbered page, inserted between p. 299 and 300 in the copy kept in the Library of the Dept. of Asian Studies, L'Orientale University, Naples). Morphologically unclear; however, a similar case of an agentive from the past stem could be *šitk* 'murderer' from *šāy- : šitt-* 'to kill'.

plant, the *Salvadora persica*, traditionally used by people in the Middle East and Central Asia in order to clean one's teeth. The "*miswā́k*-finger" could lay emphasis on the common human practice of using one's own forefinger to clean one's own teeth after eating. However, this Pšt. label might also be explained in a different way.

As we have seen above, the finger's shape, which makes it resembling to a stick, twig, sprig, etc., is perceived as one of its peculiar features and has favoured the creation of figurative expressions for 'finger' having the botanic domain as their conceptual source. In this perspective, one may also consider Eastern Pšt. *šinyáṭa* (*gúta*) 'forefinger' (also 'first toe' in RAVERTY 1860), as derived from *šinyáṭ*, 'unripe (*šin*) cereals'.

6. Equating the forefinger to a straight, pointed object is not common. However, the existence of a naming pattern based on this association is proved by a few examples we can find in some languages.[213] To them, one may associate Wx. *čuk yaŋgl* (LORIMER 1958), which could be interpreted as 'the finger standing erect'; cf. *čuk, cuq* 'erect'.[214]

If one considers Oss. Dig. '*ycht*' (i.e. *uxt*; POTT 1847: 287) as a misprint and instead read '*ychst*' (i.e. *uxst* 'spit'; TAKAZOV 2003), one could also add here Oss. Dig. *uxst ængulze*, lit. 'spit (*uxst*) – finger' (POTT: Spiessfinger), for which, however, I have only found POTT's quotation.

7. Similarly to the thumb (cf. above p. 114), the forefinger is accredited with a "regal" nature.[215] Zefr. *šō-üŋgülī* 'forefinger' bears witness to it. MAYER 1910 and GILBERTSON 1925 record Bal. *šāhmurdān* 'forefinger'; I have not found any confirmation of this label among Bal. speakers, but there is no reason to doubt its being (or having been) used somewhere in EBal.

Should we also have to assume a (unrecorded) *šāh-panǰa* 'forefinger' in Badaxšāni, where the middle finger is called *šāh-panǰa-i kalān*, lit. 'a big *šāh-panǰa*'?[216]

---

[213] Cf. VEENKER 1981: 373. For instances in Dravidian, see DED^2 2658 [3086].

[214] To the etymological references quoted in STEBLIN-KAMENSKIJ 1999: 115, add the following: Lo. *čok*, in *čok kerde* 'to straighten', *čokel* 'thin piece of wood which suddenly, like a nail, enters in someone's hand or foot or dress', (Bālā-Gar.) *čuk kirda* 'to prick up (the ears)', *čukal* 'twig', Dezf. *čok* 'erect, straight', *čokak* 'to stand up straight', and perhaps also Bal. and Br. *ǰik* 'upright, on end' (cf. ROSSI 1979: E73), Jir.-Kahn. *ǰek* 'id.' (said of hair or any other projecting or raised thing).

[215] On the forefinger as a 'Hauptfinger' see also VEENKER 1981: 369.

[216] See below p. 136.

8. As regards the fingers' sequence order, the forefinger is perceived as "the first finger" in Balochi and Minābi; cf. Bal. (Nal) *awlī lankuk* and (Mari) *sarī moṛdaγān*, lit. 'the initial finger'), Min. *kelenč avvalin* (G. BARBERA p.c.). Khot. *paḍausya haṃguṣṭi* 'the first finger' (BAILEY 1979: 50 s.v. *kaṇaiska*), an idiom containing the adjective *paḍausya* from *paḍā-* 'first', shows the same order perception.

A reversed counting direction is illustrated by the forefinger names that describe it as the fourth finger, and in particular Gz. *engulī čōram* (ŽUKOVSKIJ 1922: 110), Ydγ. *čoromī oguščiko, čaraŋgušč*; cf. Prs. *čahār* 'four', *čahārom* 'fourth' and cognates.

9. When one takes into account the collocation of a finger, one may refer to its ordinal ranking or point to its position in comparison with that of another finger. Even in the latter case, different approaches may be accounted for.

The forefinger may be described as "the finger next to the thumb".[217] Instances are Bohr. *eŋgüš palü̆-šaste* and (E)Bal. *ḍeba duhmī murdān*, provided to me by a Balochi speaker of the Mari area,[218] both meaning 'forefinger'. All this increases the probabilities that Sgd. *p(š)'nršk'*, immediately following *n(r)šk'* 'thumb' in a list of body parts and literally meaning 'behind the thumb' (SUNDERMANN 2002: 144, no. 61), may be taken as one of the Sgd. names of the forefinger, as already suggested (even if with many doubts; cf. fn. 75) by SUNDERMANN.

Yzγ. *kəranai γʷax̌t* refers to both 'forefinger' and 'ring finger', describing them as 'lateral (*kərana*)' fingers. Laterality is a feature that forefinger and ring finger share when the middle finger acts as the point of reference.

In the *Frahang-i Ōīm*, ch. X, immediately after the sequence which provides the Av. and Phl. words for 'finger' (173 *ərəzu 'ngwst*), and before the sequence mentioning the 'nail' (175 *frauāxš slwb' cygwn n'hwn*), one reads what follows: *arazān frārāzān pyš W 'ḤR 'ngwst* (174). The interpretation of this graphic string presents problems of different level: (1) the meaning of

---

[217] An equivalent expression is Lat. *pollici proximus* '(the one) near the thumb' (POTT 1847: 289, VEENKER 1981: 374 with literature).

[218] Bal. *duhmī* (as Prs. *dovvom*) does not only mean 'second' but also 'next, another'; cf. e.g. *duhmī roč/rož* 'the next day, the day after'. The usage of words for 'second' with the sense of 'next' is attested in other Iranian languages, as well.

the words in Avestan garb (*arazān frārāzān*); (2) the exact reference of the Phl. words (*<pyš W 'ḤR 'ngwst>*, /pēš u pas angust/).

In JAMASPJI – HAUG 1867: 51, *arazân frârâdhân,* considered as Av. words, and their Phl. 'equivalents' (*angušt âkhar va pēš*) are interpreted as the names of two specific fingers, i.e. the forefinger and the little finger. REICHELT (1901: 125) rules out the Avestan origin of the first two words («arazān frārazān sind Pazandwörter») and attributes to the Phl. translations (*pēš u pas angust*) the meaning of 'vorderer und hinterer Finger'. However, he gives no clues about which would be the 'vorderer' and the 'hinterer' fingers, nor a suggestion for the possible source of the Pazānd forms. In any case, *arazān frārāzān* did not find any collocation in BARTHOLOMAE 1904.

From the Av. expression in Phl. disguise, KLINGENSCHMITT (1968: 64–65) reconstructs the dvanda construction **ərəzu frārəzu** 'Finger und vorderer Teil des Fingers'. His reasoning is convincing as far as the Avestan side is concerned. It probably also fits the Phl. counterpart *pēš u pas angust,* which could be intended as 'the fore and the back part of the finger'. However, such a categorization sounds a bit strange and one could wonder which would be the salience of the back part of a finger. An alternative could be solving the sequence into *pēš angust* and *pas angust* and intending them as denominations for specific fingers. If so, which would be the fingers referred to? ABRAMJAN (1965: 5) records *axar angušt* as 'little finger'. But there is enough evidence that, should have existed a Phl. designation *pas angust*, this should have been a name for the ring finger, and not the little finger (see below p. 146). No forefinger names similar in structure to *pēš angust* are recorded in any Iranian languages, as far as I know. But Phl. *pēš angust,* if actually a finger name, could have been one of the names of the forefinger. In this case, Phl. *pēš angust* : *pas angust* might only be explained taking the middle finger as the point of reference. This hypothesis, however, needs to be supported with more valid arguments; one should also explain why only two of the five fingers have been considered as worthy of mention in the *Frahang-i Ōīm.*

10. As we have seen above with regard to Yzγ. *kəranai γ^{w}ax̌t*, Yzγ. *cəldůri γ^{w}ax̌t* is used to name both forefinger and ring finger.[219] If one compares these two fingers with the middle finger, one realizes that the formers are both 'smaller (*cəldůr*)'[220] in length and thickness. Should one reconsider in

[219] See also SKÖLD 1936: 186; GAUTHIOT 1916: 254 fn. 1 («l'index et l'annulaire s'appellent tous deux *cəldūr wax̌t* 'petit doigt'»).

[220] On Yzγ. *cəldůr* 'small(er), young(er)' see below, p. 155 fn. 269.

this perspective Makrāni Bal. *kasānen* (?) 'forefinger' quoted in MORGENSTIERNE 1932a: 40, with which I did away elsewhere (FILIPPONE 2000–2003: 78 n. 41), treating it as a misunderstanding? Bal. *kasān* 'little' is actually used, together with the word for 'finger' and *never alone*, to name the little finger (see below p. 159). If it is really used somewhere in Makrān with reference to the forefinger, *kasānen* should in any case be followed by the relevant word for 'finger'.

Possibly, to the forefinger's relative dimension also points Pšt. *bónḍa gúta* 'forefinger'. It could be explained as containing a form related to *bunḍ* 'short; cut-off'.

The forefinger's relative dimension motivates other forefinger names. However, in a stark contrast with those we have seen above, Lārest. *kelike gotû*,[221] Sed. *uŋgulī-bale*, Yγn. *kátta pánǰa*[222] (*kátta páx(x)a* XROMOV 1972),[223] and doubtfully Semn. *masin angošt*,[224] all describe the forefinger as a "big finger".

11. Words originally meaning 'finger', without further specification, may be used to name the forefinger, exactly as it happens to the thumb (p. 117 above) and the other fingers as well (pp. 140, 148 and 169 below). To this iconomastic type, the following belong: Lār. *angošt* 'finger; finger *par excellence*, i.e. forefinger' (KAMIOKA – YAMADA 1979),[225] Keš. *aŋguš*, Voniš. *uŋguss*, Badaxš. *panǰa* 'finger; the first finger' (also 'the open hand')', Siv. *gos* (ZIĀN 1960)[226], Kāz. *penǰe* (BEHRUZI 2002; 'finger' in SALĀMI 2004), Wan. *nguṭā* 'thumb, also the first and second finger' and probably also Haz. *narxūn* (DULLING 1973).[227]

12. To conclude this review of forefinger names, it remains to mention a couple which I have not been able to analyse.

---

221 On Lārest. *got* 'big' see above, p. 101.

222 On Yγn. *pánǰa* 'the five fingers; middle finger' see below p. 140.

223 According to MIRZOZODA 2008, *katta paxxa* is both 'thumb' and 'index finger'; cf. above, p. 103 and fn. 151.

224 The data collected for Semnāni do not tally; cf. *masína* 'middle finger' in SHAKIBI-GUILANI – JAVAHERI 1993.

225 However, *angošt* is recorded as 'finger' in KAMIOKA – RAHBAR – HAMIDI 1986 and lacks in EQTEDĀRI 1955.

226 Siv. *gūs* is recorded as 'finger' in EILERS 1988 and LECOQ 1976 (*gos*). See above p. 57.

227 See above, p. 84.

These are EBal. *kušāl*, provided to me by a Bugti speaker; (dial.) Taj. *suvor*, used in the area of Vaxio-Bolo (ROZENFEL'D 1982); Mamas. *lôti*.

LECOQ 2002 records Biz. *šepoškoš* as 'forefinger'; however, the "lice-killer finger" is generally a common pattern for the thumb name (see above p. 115).

CHAPTER FIVE: THE MIDDLE FINGER

1. In all languages, including the Iranian, the middle finger names emphasize in most cases the central position of this finger as compared to the others.[228] This plain acknowledgement accounts for Av. (gen.) *maδəmahe ərəzvō*, MPrs. *miyānag angust*, which have already been commented above,[229] Sgd. *miδānč angušt*, occurring in P 14, the same Buddhist text in which *mazēx angušt* 'thumb' and *niwēδēne-angušt* 'forefinger'[230] also occur, as well as all the Modern Ir. labels for 'middle finger' that will be listed in what follows.

These are Prs. *angošt-e miāne/miāni/miānin* (MOKRI 2005: 264), Taj. *angušt-i miona*, dial. Taj. (Darvāz, Kara-Tegin) *lik-i mina* (ROZENFEL'D 1982), Bxt. *keliče miune* (my own data), Lārest. *kelike-mûna*, Gil. *meyoni angušt*, Semn. *miyonin angošt*, Šahm. *miyon angošt*, Lāsg. *miyonin engošt*, Zefr. *üŋgüli meyū*, Bohr. *eŋgüš mühǖna*, Sed. *uŋgulī-miyūn(ī)*, etc. In EIr., one finds Pšt. *myándza gúta*, Ōrm. *mənzaŋgušt*, Par. *(angušt-e) myanakåli*, Ydγ. *malanë oguščigo*, Mnǰ. *malenig agūšḱa*, *mālenig* (*malanīgo āguškʸo* IIFL-II), Yzγ. *maδeni γʷaxt* (*maδīnī* GAUTHIOT 1916: 254 fn. 1), Šγn. *miδenǰ angixt* (*miδēnā angixt* and *miyůna angixt* ZARUBIN 1960), Baǰ. *miδenʒ ingaxt* and Yγn. *bidóni angúšt, bidóni činčilák, bidóni panǰá* (*bidūni paxa* XROMOV 1972).

EBal. *nīām(aγ)ī* and SBal. *tokī* (adj.) 'middle' derive respectively from *nīām* (by metathesis from *mīān*[231]) and *tok* 'centre, inside'.[232] EBal. (Mari) *nīāmaγī murdānaγ* and *nīāmī moṛdaγān*[233] shares with SBal. (Dašt) *tokī lankuk* the emphasis on the median position of this finger. However, these Bal. idioms are less used than *gaḍḍī*, the current Bal. denomination of the middle finger, notwithstanding their being perceived as more polite and educated than the latter: they are used on those occasions in which *gaḍḍī* might be considered too 'rude' (see below § 5).

---

228 A myriad of examples may be quoted from any language of the world; for a few instances see VEENKER 1981: 370.

229 See pp. 95 ff., also for a possible different interpretation ("middle-seized finger") of both phrases.

230 See above p. 97 and p. 123.

231 In the Ir. *miān*-family, further cases of metathesis are recorded; cf. e.g. Sist. *nmō*, Āmor. *ni'om* (*niyum* MOQDAM 1949: 90), etc.

232 Probably a semantic extension from an original 'valley'; cf. FILIPPONE 1996: 340–341.

233 *nyāmayi murdān* (?) 'forefinger' in MORGENSTIERNE 1932a: 40 comes from a misfiling by MORGENSTIERNE of DAMES' *Glossary* (where it correctly appears as 'middle finger').

CENTRE is often verbalized in Iranian by means of lexical processes (semantic change or derivation) based on metaphorical associations with body parts whose position is perceived as central, according to a strategy which may be considered as a universal. The waist is one of these parts. Prs. *miān* (and cognates) 'middle' probably originated in this way.[234] Similarly, Oss. *astæw* 'waist; loins' has acquired the sense of 'centre, middle'.[235] The derived adjective *astæwkkag* 'middle' occurs in the Oss. middle finger name, which is *astæwkkag ængwylʒ* (my own data).

Other body parts which have been involved in similar processes are the heart and the navel.[236]

HEART is the metaphorical source for CENTRE in (Gor.) Gahwārai; cf. *dilî-râs* 'middle', with *dil* 'heart' and *râs* belonging to Prs. *rāst* 'right' and cognates, many of which have acquired the additional meaning of 'direction, side'; see Prs. *rāstā*, Šir. *rāsse* (SAMANDAR 1999: 128), Hanǰ. *rās*, Vfs. *yek-rasd, yey-ras* ('straight to, directly to') and further references in CHRISTENSEN – BARR 1939: 322. Gor. (Gahw.) *dilî-râs* occurs in the lexicalized phrase *kilik-i dilî-râsin* 'middle finger'.

NAVEL is the metaphorical source for many Kurdish nominals (nouns and adjectives) connected to the notion of CENTRE ('(the) middle; (the) inside'):[237] see KurmKrd. *nav, navçe, navîn, nîv, naverast* etc., (ᶜAmādiya) *nav* 'centre (rare), milieu', *nîv* 'half, centre, milieu', (Jabal Sinǰār) *nêv, nîv* 'milieu, centre' (BLAU 1975), SouthKrd. *nâv, nâw, nâvî, nêvî, nâvîn, nâwig, nâwr̲âs, nêwar̲âs, nêwar̲âst, nêwân*, (Mahâb.) *nēw, nēwân, nēwarâst*, (Krmnš.) *nâw*, (Garr.) *nāårâs* 'middle'. Obviously, Krd. *–ras/-râs* belong to the same *rāst-*'direction' group we have seen above.

In Iranian, the NAVEL = CENTRE equation may be illustrated by further examples. Even Prs. *nāf* is used in the sense of 'centre', though seemingly mostly in association with specific collocates (*nāf-e biābān* 'the middle of the desert'; *nāf-e dašt* 'the middle of the country/desert'; *dar nāf-e šahr* 'in

---

234 Cf. Av. *maiδyāna-, maiδyąna-* «'Mitte'; a) des Leibes […] Ableit. aus ¹*maiδya-*»; ¹*maiδya-* « I) Adj. […] 'medius', zeitlich; […] 2) m., n. 'Mitte […] insbes. des Leibes, 'Taille') » (BARTHOLOMAE 1904).

235 Oss. *astæw* is also used as a postposition with a locative function ('in middle of, inside'); cf. IESOJ s.v.

236 For the 'heart' → 'centre' shifting see FILIPPONE 1996: 307, with a few Ir. examples (to which add Tāl. (Māsule) *dela* 'dedans', LAZARD 1979); for the 'navel' → 'centre' shifting see also Skt. (RV) *nā́bhi-* 'Nabel; Mittelpunkt' (EWA II: 11).

237 Note that KurmKrd. *nav* has also acquired the meaning of 'waist'.

the middle of the town', etc.).[238] Kerm. *nāf,* Arāk. *nâf,* Xor. *nāv* (ADIB TUSI 1963–1964) may also be used with the sense of 'the middle'.

The centrality of the *nav*-series as 'middle; inside' in the Kurdish lexicon has favoured a lexicalization process which has produced a few *nav*-derivatives as the most current nouns for 'navel'; cf. Kurm. *nav(ik), nêw(ik)*, SouthKrd. *nâv(ik), nâwik(a), nêvik, nêwik* 'navel'.

Kurdish and Lakki labels for 'middle finger' are: KurmKrd. *tilîya navîn, tilîya nêvî* (*tilya navê* KURDOEV 1960), SouthKrd. *dipilâ nêvakî* (EBRĀHIMPUR 1994b s.v. *angošt*), Mukri *qâmîk î nêwê* (also 'ring finger'), Bābā-Krd. *kámki nīū rāst,* Garr. *kelik e nāârâs,* Lak. *keľek nomen.*

Bast. *angošt mârkā* is the Bast. name of the middle finger. It contains *mârkā* 'middle', an adjective widespread in Lārestāni; cf. Lār., Ger. *mâreka* 'middle, in the middle'.

As a formal alternative to *angošt-e miān(-e/-i)*, Persian has *angošt-e vasati*, with *vasati* 'middle', an ancient, well integrated Ar. loanword. Ar. *al-wusṭá* 'middle finger' has been borrowed in Persian, as well: cf. Prs. *vostā* (also MOINFAR 1981: 230) and Taj. *angušt-i vusto.* KurmKrd. *orte* 'middle, centre' is a Turkish loanword; KurmKrd. *tilîya ortê* 'middle finger' parallels Turk. *ortaparmak* 'id.'.

It seems reasonable to interpret Haz. *narxūn-i-γulgina* 'middle toe' (DULLING 1973), but with all probability also 'middle finger',[239] as 'the finger/toe of the middle', connecting *γulgina* to Haz. *γōl* 'middle, centre' (< Mong. *γoul*), and rejecting DULLING's suggestion («? perh. *γulgina* < Tu. '*qol*' (= hand) & dimin. suffix. '*-gina*'»).

2. Khot. *śą haṃguṣṭi* (BAILEY 1979: 50 s.v. *kaṇaiska*) 'middle finger' (lit. 'the second finger') takes into account the sequence of the fingers in an ordinal ranking. Khot. *śą* means 'second', and being second is what happens to the middle finger when one starts to count from the forefinger. In a similar way, the middle finger is called *kelenče dovvom* (lit. 'the second finger') in Minābi (G. BARBERA p.c.).

---

[238] This usage is considered "familiar" by LAZARD 1990a; according to ᶜAli Ašraf SĀDEQI (p.c.), however, *nāf* as 'middle' is archaic, being mostly found in the old phases of New Persian.

[239] Since fingers and toes are not lexically differentiated in Iranian, any differentiation found in dictionaries may be ascribed to a projection by the editor of his own conceptual categories. Particularly odd is the meaning 'middle toe' attributed to *narxūn-i-γulgina* as confronted with the etymology doubtfully advanced by DULLING 1973.

3. The middle finger is undoubtedly the longest among the fingers, while in thickness it is second only to the thumb, which is, on its part, very short. For this reason, as already stated above (p. 95), the middle finger shares with the thumb the "the big(gest) finger" label type,[240] and this fact may create a large rate of ambiguity, which sometimes only the context may help to remove. Prs. *angošt-e bozorg* means both 'thumb' and 'middle finger'; EBal. (Nāsirābād) *mazanẽ angrī* 'thumb' parallels W/SBal. *mazanẽ lankuk* 'thumb' (see above p. 97); Yzγ. *qəldůri γ°ax̌t* is given as 'middle finger' in ĖDEL'MANN 1971 and 'thumb' in GAUTHIOT 1916 and SKÖLD 1936 (see above p. 107). Similarly, (South.) Krd. *âl, yâḻ* is 'middle finger' in HAŽĀR 1990, EBRĀHIMPUR 1994a and 'thumb' in EBRĀHIMPUR 1994b (cf. *âl*, s.v. *angošt*).[241] Fluctuation in meaning is attested for Sgd. *mazēx angušt*, as well. Since it occurs in two different passages where the names of other fingers are mentioned, we are allowed to assume that it means 'thumb' in P 14 and 'middle finger' in the body-parts list published by SUNDERMANN (2002: 144 no. 58; see also above p. 97).

The middle finger is depicted as "the big (finger)" by the following idioms: Prs. *angošt-e mehin* (DEHX),[242] (dial.) Taj. *čilik-i kalon* (KALBĀSI 1995), Lo. *kalak-e buzorg* (UNVALA 1958: 14), Gz. *engolī-bäle,*[243] Abiā. *angöšta görde.*[244] Semn. *masína* is given as 'middle finger' in SHAKIBI-GUILANI – JAVAHERI 1993[245] and as 'forefinger' (*masin angošt*) in SOTUDE 1963; see above p. 131.

Badaxš. *šāh-panǰa-i kalān* 'middle finger' deserves a few comments. What is defined here as big (*kalān*) is not a finger in general, but a *šāh-panǰa*, for which the meaning 'forefinger' has been suggested above, p. 128. If so, the relative dimension of this finger is not evaluated taking into account the whole fingers, but only two of them (both recognized as "regal", *šāh-*). And the middle finger is surely bigger than the forefinger.

---

240 The middle finger as a 'big(ger) finger' is also found in other languages; compare for instance Fr. *majeur* 'middle finger'.

241 On the possible interpretation of SouthKrd. *âl* as 'the big one', see above, p. 110.

242 On Prs. *mehin* see above p. 98.

243 The *bale*-type for 'big, large' is an isogloss delimiting a south-central grouping in the Central Plateau dialect area (southeastern Kāšāni dialects and Esfahāni dialects) (KRAHNKE 1976: 215–217, and Map V – 28). As for the etymology of Gz. *bäli, bälẽ*, EILERS (1979 s.v.) advances two alternatives: (1) < SW **barda-* (NW **barza-*) 'high'; (2) < SW **vardak* (< *vazr̥ka-*, with metathesis). STILO (2007: 108) supports the latter.

244 On Abiā. *görd* and the *gord*-type 'big' see also above pp. 103 f.

245 On Semn. *masin* 'big' see above p. 98.

The middle finger is simply depicted as a "regal finger", without further considerations, in Kargānrudi, a central Tāleši variety, where it is called *šo angəšta* (D. GUIZZO, p.c.).

4. To remove any possible ambiguity which a general reference to bigness may create, one may stress upon the middle finger's relevant dimension, i.e. length. This is what happens with Prs. *angošt-e derāz*, (dial.) Taj. *čilik-i daroz* (KALBĀSI 1995), Gz. *engolī dirāz* and KurmKrd. *tilîya dirêj* (RIZGAR 1993), which have Engl. *long finger* 'middle finger' as their equivalent.

The appropriate usage of words belonging to the DIMENSION domain is in some way contingent on different alternatives of space and shape categorization inside any specific conceptual and cultural system. The question is complicated and goes beyond the aims of this book. The following scanty considerations, mainly focussed on Balochi, may be useful to our reasoning on the middle finger denominations.

In Balochi, the upright position of any object is a prerequisite for its vertical dimension to be recognized as *burzī* ('height') and for the same object to be, in case, recognized as *burz* ('high / tall'). However, it is not a binding condition. In fact, the vertical dimension is often identified as *drāǰī*, which commonly refers to a horizontal dimension ('length'). This does not mean that Bal. *drāǰī* and *burzī* with reference to the vertical dimension are semantically equivalent. When using *burzī* (or the adjective *burz*), one is not providing any information about the object's shape, the considered dimension and the proportion between all the object dimensions, all factors which on the contrary condition the usage of *drāǰī* (and *drāǰ*). The vertical dimension of a three-dimensional object may be identified as *drāǰī* in the following cases: (1) the object is perceived as having a "controllable height" (with which I mean the possibility for human people, taking their body as a reference point, of "controlling" it), provided that it is not marked by another dimension perceived as more salient; (2) though having an "uncontrollable height", the object has a tapering shape, such as, e.g., that of a lamp-post. The use of *drāǰī* when speaking of the human body height is absolutely frequent and areally unmarked in Balochi.

Prs. *derāz(i)* and cognates do not behave differently from Bal. *drāǰ(ī)*. Consequently, the names of the middle finger listed above may describe it both as 'long' and as 'tall'; in the latter case, the evoked image would be that of a standing up finger, similar to a little fellow. This could be the case with SouthKrd. *dôla dirêž* 'middle finger'(EBRĀHIMPUR 1994a, SAFIZĀDE 2001), if one interprets the head of this lexicalized phrase as *dôl* 'child, offspring'; see also Kurm. *dol* 'seed, sperm; breed; descendents, offspring, progeny' (CHYET 2003: < Turk.).

Similarly to the expressions containing *derāz*-cognates, Taj. *angušt-i raso* 'middle finger' may be interpreted both as a descriptive and a figurative expression, since *raso* means both 'long' and 'tall'. To the figurative pattern that lays emphasis on the finger's "tallness", belong Prs. *angošt-e boland*, Gz. *engolī-biländ*, SulKrd. *ba̱laberze*, SouthKrd. (Krmnš.) *bâ̱lâ barza*, (cf. SouthKrd. *bâlâberz* 'tall'). SOTUDE 1986 attributes Nāi. *qabābilandu* 'middle finger' to the child language; even in this idiom the reference to tallness is evident, but I do not know how to interpret *qabā*.

In Gazi the middle finger, equated to a reputable, tall man, is also labelled *abo bulend* (ŽUKOVSKIJ 1922: 110); to him, the appellative *abo*, a well known Semitic loanword (cf. Ar. *abū* 'father', etc.), has been reserved.

To this humanized finger one might also ascribe a proper name. The Zoroastrians of Yazd call their middle finger *hasan dirāz* (VAHMAN – ASATRIAN 2002: 59), lit. 'Hasan, the tall', a name which parallels SBšk. (Garu) *hasan bolan* (G. BARBERA p.c.). Even an ethnic identity may be granted to this finger, as illustrated by *tork(e) boland* 'the tall Turk', an alternative to *hasan boland* in the NBšk. dialects spoken in Sardašt (G. BARBERA p.c.). The choice of Hasan as the middle finger's personal name is not casual: being a very frequent name, it is often used to refer to paradigmatic characters having specific peculiarities. In Zarqāni, *hasan* is the name with which thieves address each other, or with which one addresses a thief, even when one knows the thief's name; *hasan-e bozorg* means 'the head of the thieves'. In Širāzi, *hasan-e gap* is used with exactly the same sense. In an Argot Prs. dictionary (SAMĀI 2003), *hasan* is given as 'countryman', or as 'townsman with the education and culture of a countryman', or simply as 'stupid person'. Stupidity is just one of the features which human people sometimes attribute to their middle finger, as we will see below, § 7.

5. The middle finger is the only finger that is named with one and the same word all over the Bal. dialectal areas, with the only exclusion of Karachi. It is currently referred to as *gaḍḍī*, which may or not be followed by the word for 'finger' current in each particular dialectal area (viz., *lankuk, hor* or *murdayān*). The Bal. labels quoted above (EBal. *mazanẽ angrī,* lit. 'the big finger', EBal. *nīāmayī murdānay,* SBal. *tokī lankuk*, lit. 'the middle finger'), iconomastic types based on the middle finger's size and position, are only

possible alternatives, sometimes considered as more appropriate since they better meet the social expectations, especially in very formal situations.

The peculiarity of Bal. *gaḍḍī* consists in its being to a certain extent a taboo word, so that uttering or hearing it may cause a special reaction, such as a laughing up one's sleeve or a lowering of the tone of one's voice. The fact is that it immediately evokes images bound to the domain of sexuality and/or obscenity. This word, seemingly of Indian origin, is probably borrowed from Sindhi; cf. Si. *gaḍḍi* '(slang) thrusting one's finger up the fundament', which could be related to **gaḍḍ-*[1] 'dig, bury', and **gaḍḍa-* 'hole, pit' (CDIAL 3979 and 3981). However, no IA word for 'middle finger' resembling Bal. *gaḍḍī* is found, as far as I know. Br. *gaḍḍī* 'middle finger' (see also *gaḍḍī kanning* 'to stuff up (obsc.)' BRAY 1934) is possibly a Bal. loanword.

On the conceptual equation FINGER = MALE GENITAL ORGAN and the connection between sexuality and fingers denominations we have already spoken above (see p. 45). In most Bal. areas, sticking up the middle finger or bending it downwards while keeping straight forwards the other fingers, one transmits obscene messages: cf. *gaḍḍī kanag* 'to stick one's finger up (either physically poking someone from behind with the middle finger, or sticking this finger in the air as a sign of abuse. Very impolite)' and by semantic extension, 'to fiddle with, to mess with' (RAZZAQ –BUKSH – FARRELL 2001). In a few areas of Balochistan, however, one may transmit the same message using the thumb. This explains the fact that the Karachi Bal. speakers (and probably a few EBal. speakers) name their thumb *gaḍḍī.*[246] Karachi Bal. *gaḍḍī pešdārag* (RAZZAQ – BUKSH – FARRELL 2001) and EBal. *ḍeb ḍassaγ* (MĪṬHĀ – SURAT 1960)[247] exactly correspond to Ur. *angūtā dikhānā* 'to show the thumb', i.e. 'to signify a desire for sexual intercourse' and, metaphorically, 'to give a refusal, to answer rudely' (PLATTS 1930).

A further instance of name alternation between middle finger and thumb, emphasizing the close conceptual relationship between these two fingers, is Bal. *dīp* 'middle finger', quoted in ELFENBEIN 1990-II and DAMES 1891. Bal. *dīp* seems to be a phonetic variant (a different recording?) of EBal. *deb/ḍeb* 'thumb'.[248] However, no EBal. speaker confirmed to me such a usage of *deb/ḍeb*, nor have I found any occurrences of it in published texts.

---

[246] Also *gaḍḍīẽ lankuk* (RAZZAQ – BUKSH – FARRELL 2001). For EBal., see MAYER 1910 (s.v. finger) *gadī* 'thumb' (unknown to my EBal. informants).

[247] On EBal. *ḍeb* 'thumb' see above, p. 119.

[248] Differently, DAMES (1891) distinguishes *deb* 'thumb' from *dīp* 'middle finger'.

6. Middle finger names deriving through a semantic restriction from words originally meaning 'finger' are the following: Wan. *nguṭā* (also 'thumb and first finger') and Yγn. *pánǰa* in Eastern Iranian; Keš. *aŋguš* and Voniš. *uŋguss* in the Central Dialect area; Sist. *āngol*, Lār. *kelike angol* (KAMIOKA – YAMADA 1979) and Min. *angol* (G. BARBERA p.c.) in South-East Iran. It is not excluded that the *angol*-type middle fingers may evoke the same obscene implications as Bal. *gaḍḍī.*[249]

Roš. *lakak iŋgaxt* (SKÖLD 1936: 186) 'middle finger' is likely to be connected with the terms for 'finger' found in a few Tajik dialects, i.e. *lik, likak* etc. we have seen above, p. 62.

7. MAYER (1910) and GILBERTSON (1925 s.v. *finger*) provide *nizānaγī murdān* as one of the EBal. names of the middle finger. MORGENSTIERNE (1932a: 40) also quotes it. None of them tries to explain this idiom, of which I have found no occurrences, either in oral or in written texts. Bal. *nizānaγ* as an isolated word is unattested and its meaning was unknown to the Bal. speakers I asked about. We can only try to advance a hypothetical derivation.

In Balochi finger-rhymes, the middle finger is said to be *ganok* ('fool, foolish, unwise'). The following are two instances of that kind of rhymes with five lines, where each line is devoted to one of the fingers:

(a)		(b)	
thumb	*šast ki mast*	little f.	*čunkī čulankī*
foref.	*kāsag-līsok*	ring f.	*zarrānī bānuk*
middle f.	*gaḍḍī ganok*	middle f.	*gaḍḍī ganok int*
ring f.	*zarrānī bānok*	Foref.	*kāsag čaṭṭit*
little f.	*čičkul mačkul*	thumb	*drustānī māt int*

The main difference between these two rhymes is the reverse order: (a), which I have collected from Ir. Bal. speakers from Sarāwān,[250] starts from the thumb, while (b), published in SAYYAD HASHMI 2000 s.v. *čunkī*, starts from the little finger and ends with the thumb, said *drustānī māt*, i.e. 'the mother of all'. The middle finger's *ganok*-nature has been confirmed to me by several Baloch.

---

[249] Cf. for example Sist. *āngol kardā*, Rod. *angol*, Lir.-Dil. *angûl(ak) dâdan*, etc. All of them refer to real or figurative obscene senses and are used as a kind of abuse.

[250] The syntactic construction of *zarrānī bānok* (for which see below, p. 143), opposite to the usual one in Sarāwāni Balochi, suggests that this little rhyme did not originate in Sarāwān.

Another EBal. term for 'foolish, ignorant' is *nāzānox,* which MAYER (1910) provides together with *nādān/nāδān*, a Prs. loanword; cf. Prs. *nādān* 'foolish person, fool, unlearned'. Similar forms, with slight differences at the morphological level, are *nāzant, bezānt, nābizānt* (SAYYAD HASHMI 2000), *nă̄zant* (BARKER – MENGAL 1969), *nāzānt* (ELFENBEIN 1990-II) etc. All of them are composed by the negative prefix, *nă̄*-, plus the present stem *zān/(dān)*- 'to know, to be wise' (or the past stem *–zānt*) plus (as for *nāzānok/x*) the agentive suffix *-ok/x*. As for meaning, they all may implicate a lack of knowledge and a lack of experience (from 'innocent, naive', to 'ignorant', 'stupid', 'fool' etc.). Cognate forms in other Ir. languages are commented on in SKJÆRVØ 1975: 121.

However, *nizānayī* is not *nazānayī*, and the *-i-* vowel remains unexplained,[251] unless one assumes that *ni-* in MAYER 1910 is a misprint for *na-* (what is absolutely possible); GILBERTSON (1925) may have taken this expression directly from MAYER 1910, like MORGENSTIERNE (1932a) certainly has. Should this be the case, *nizānayī murdān* in MAYER 1910 would stay for *nazānayī murdān* and mean 'the finger of the foolishness/ignorance', a quite befitting label for a finger that in Balochi folklore is commonly treated as a *ganok*. But all this remains a guesswork for now.

Just as the middle finger is considered as stupid and simple-minded by Baloch, it is depicted as "the big naïf" or "the big without fruit" by the Maghrebine people, as may be inferred from children rhymes published in CHEBEL 1999: 88–89. The same prejudice against this finger might motivate SouthKrd. *zarnaquta, zirnaquta* 'middle finger; small, unfledged sparrow', Krmnš. *zaranaquta* 'middle finger'. KURDOEV (1960) gives *zerneqûte* as a SouthKrd. word, meaning 'nestling' and 'greenhorn': we may recognize here the same metaphorical association which has produced the different senses [(1) young bird; (2) unexperienced person] of Engl. *fledgling*.

8. Wan. *lakó lakə́ṛ* 'middle finger' (ELFENBEIN 1984), recorded in Pashto as 'ring finger' (see *lākúlakā́ṛa* below, p. 148), shares with Xur. *sozåboland* 'middle finger', lit. 'the high grass', the conceptual connection to the botanic domain.

[251] I have found no *ni-* instead of the negative prefix *na-* in any published Bal. texts (nor have I any information of a verb in Balochi or any other Ir. languages composed of *dān-/zān-* ('to know') plus the prefix *ni-*).

9. To conclude, the following middle finger names remain unexplained: Abiā. *kūreqor'ōxōne*; KurmKrd. *tilîya daradûmê* (RIZGAR 1993); SorKrd. *qamkî he<u>l</u>me tûte* (KURDOEV – JUSUPOVA 1983).

CHAPTER SIX: THE RING FINGER

1. There is a lot of ring finger names in a large amount of languages which lay emphasis on the custom of putting rings on this finger. Engl. *ring finger* illustrates this much productive iconomastic pattern perfectly.[252]

Prs. *angošt-e halqe* (LAZARD 1990a) and *angošt-e angoštar* (ĀRYĀNPUR KĀŠĀNI 1979, s.v. *ring finger*) 'ring finger' contrast each other in that an Ar. loanword (*halqe*) alternates with an original Prs. word (*angoštar*(*i*)), but both literally mean 'the finger of the ring'. Correspondently, Tajik has *angušt-i halqa* and *angušt-i anguštarī*. The same iconomastic pattern is found in Northern Kurdish, as is proved by KurmKrd. *tilîya gustîlê / gustîlkê / gustîlkirinê / hinglîskê* (*tilya gistîlê*; *pîçê gistîlê / hingilîskê* AMÎRXAN 1992).

The Bal. labels *mundrīke lankuk* and *čallaī* 'ring finger', both recorded in Iranian Balochistan (respectively in Kasarkand and Irānšahr), explicitly mention the ring, *mundrī(k/g)* (also *mundīk* SAYAD HASHMI 2000) and *čalla* (also *čallaw*, *čallo*). The former is an IA lw. (< Si. *munḍrī* 'ring', GEIGER 1890–1891: 455) and is current in EBal. and SBal. (not only EHB, as stated in ELFENBEIN 1990-II). The latter is mainly used in WBal. and has cognates in Eastern Persian and EIr. languages; cf. AfγPrs. *čilla* 'finger-ring without stone; ear-ring', Her. *čalla* 'ear-ring', Sist. *čalla* 'lock of hair; etc.', Pšt. *čalá* 'ear-ring', Išk. *čīl(l)a* (*čelik* IIFL II), Šγn. *čil(l)ā* 'finger-ring', etc. It has been considered as an IA lw. (cf. Hi. *čhallā*, Si. *chəlo*, *chəla*, also ROSSI 1979: I32 for Br. *čallaw* 'ring').

Most of the Bal. names for the ring finger emphasize the metal rings are commonly made of, i.e. gold (Bal. *zarr*). In all Bal. varieties the ring finger is named *zarrī*, possibly followed by the word for 'finger' (i.e., *zarrī lankuk* and *zarrī murdāna*[g]) or *zardānag* (Noške, i.e. 'the one having gold'). And since wearing jewels among Baloch is traditionally a habit of women, especially of women of a high status, the finger which rings are used to be put on is equated to a fair, jewelled lady: this finger becomes nothing less than a *zarrānī bānok* (Noške, Xarān, Sarāwān, Karachi). Considering the derivation with the suffix *-ak*, one may attribute to Br. *zarak* 'third finger', an Ir. source other than Balochi (see ROSSI 1979: F172). The data at my disposal, however, do not allow the identification of this hypothetical source, since I

252 For a few examples of the "ring-finger" and "gold-finger" patterns in languages other than Iranian, see VEENKER 1981: 370–371; BENNETT 1982: 13 ff.

have found no "gold-finger" in other Ir. languages; the source could also have been a Bal. variety not yet described.

To the habit of wearing a ring (more specifically, the engagement ring) on this finger also points Lār. *kelike nāmzadi* (KAMIOKA – YAMADA 1979), lit. 'the finger of the engagement'; it is also possible, however, that this name evokes different practices symbolizing the engagement (not necessarily involving the ring finger), which are unknown to me.

2. In a very large, substantially contiguous geographic area, where languages from different linguistic families are spoken, such as Finno-Ugric and Balto-Slavonic, Southern Caucasian, Turkish, Mongolian, Uralic and Tibetan, the ring finger does not have any name, or, better to say, its same name depicts it is a 'finger without a name'.[253] Also in Sanskrit one finds *ánāmā-* and *ánāmikā-* 'ring finger', male nominals from *ánāman-* 'nameless; infamous'; I am not aware of the existence of similar forms in any modern IA languages, though.[254]

Prs. *binām* 'ring finger' (lit. '(the one) without a name') is recorded in traditional dictionaries (DEHX), but is completely unfamiliar to Prs. speakers of Iran, as I could notice in my fieldwork. "Nameless" ring fingers are Taj. *angušt-i benom*, KurmKrd. *tilya bênav* (RIZGAR 1993) and Oss. *œnœnom œngwylʒ* (my own data).

Why should the ring finger be a "nameless finger"? [255] Different answers have been given to this question. The most obvious explanation is that no importance has been attached to it; a sort of laziness in the creative human activity would have then encouraged the development of this label pattern, so largely spread. This is what ERDAL (1981: 123) thinks of the Turk. name of the ring finger. Another argument points to a linguistic interdiction: the ring finger could be culturally connoted in such a way that the usage of a specific name would be not recommended, since even the name alone could evoke its dangerousness. VEENKER (1981: 365) cites ERDEDI's remarks on the matter: in Finno-Ugric, such a taboo would be justified by the fact that ancient sacrificial practices used to require blood flow from the ring finger. A similar hypothesis had been already suggested

[253] Cf. also VEENKER 1981: 365.

[254] POTTS 1847: 284 quotes a similar Hi. expression (from ADAM).

[255] Note that one may consider in this light even the lacking of a name, as is the case with Garrusi, where, according to CHRISTENSEN – BARR 1939: 305, there are names for all the fingers except for the ringfinger («Der Ringfinger hat keine Name»).

by POTT (1847: 297–298) with regard to Skt. *ánāmā-*; see also BENNETT 1982: 17 for the ring finger names in New High German and Swedish. Be that as it may, "the nameless finger" in Tajik, Kurdish and Ossetic could also be explained as the result of a linguistic contact (perhaps even lexical calques); "the nameless finger" pattern could have get the status of an areal lexical feature.

3.1 As far as the ring finger names grounded on the finger's position are concerned, I can only repeat what has already been said above. Different strategies for computation are attested in Iranian: if computation starts from the thumb, the ring finger actually happens to be the fourth finger, as proved by Prs. *angošt-e čahārom*; see DEHX, supported by some Prs. definitions in glossaries and dictionaries, as is the case with AFŠĀR 1989 s.v. Yzd. *angošt-e pas-kiliči* 'ring finger [*angošt-e čahārom-e dast*]'. If computation starts from the forefinger, the ring finger becomes the third finger, as illustrated by Khot. *dīda hagauṣṭa* (BAILEY 1979: 50 s.v. *kaṇaiska*), EBal. (Mari) *semī moṛdaγān,* Min. *kelenče sevvom* (G. BARBERA p.c.). If computation starts from the little finger, the ring finger will be perceived as the second finger and this counting direction accounts for Prs. (*angošt-e) dovvom* (DEHX); one finds Prs. *angošt-e dovvom* as the Prs. equivalent of Xur. *māye kleič* 'ring finger' in FARAHVAŠI 1976: 2 or Krd. *tilyâ bâbilîçk* 'id.' in SAFIZĀDE 2001.

3.2 The ring finger names that take into account the position of this finger mostly emphasize its closeness to another finger, which in most cases is the little finger. This iconomastic pattern is found in many languages, both ancient and modern: see Skt. *upa-madhyamā-* and *upa-kaniṣṭhikā-* 'the finger next to the little finger, the last finger but one', Lat. *proximus minimo digitus*, etc. (ANDRÉ 1991: 103–104; also VEENKER 1981: 371).

In Central Iran, we find Nāi. *engoli var keliču,* Zefr. *üŋgülī ver ḱasa* 'the finger near [*var/ver*] to the little [*keliču/kas*] one' and ZorYzd. *pas-kilīčōg, angošt-e pas-kiliči* (AFŠĀR 1989) '(the finger) next to/following [*pas*] the little finger [*kilīčōg/kiliči*]'.

EBal. *čīnča dumī murdānaγ* 'ring finger', lit. 'the finger next to the little finger [*čīnča*]' is the counterpart of *ḍeba duhmī murdān* 'forefinger', lit. 'the finger next to the thumb' (see above p. 129), both provided to me by a Mari speaker, while in Šuγni, where *ʒalik* and *lakak* are labels for 'little finger', *pis-ʒalik angiχ̌t*[*aθ*] and *pis-lakak angiχ̌t*[*aθ*] (ZARUBIN 1960) are 'ring finger[s]';[256] cf. Šγn. *pis* 'next, following'.

On the Paz.? (pseudo) Av.? expression *arazān frārāzān* and its Phl. translation *pēš u pas angust* in the *Frahang-i Ōīm* has been discussed above, p. 130. There, it has been hinted at the possibility that Phl. *pēš angust* and *pas angust* could refer to the forefinger and the ring finger respectively, according to a iconomastic pattern that takes the middle finger as a point of reference. The Prs. expression *angošt-e pas* found in the *Kāmel at-Taᶜbīr*, with the meaning of 'ring finger' (MOKRI 2005: 264), as well as Yzd-JPrs. *passâyi* 'ring finger', i.e. the finger following the middle finger, could support this suggestion.

Both the ring finger and the forefinger are perceived as "lateral fingers", if compared to the middle finger, to which they are next. This is proved by Yzγ. *kəranai γʷaχ̌t*, which means both 'ring finger' and 'forefinger' (see also above, p. 129).

3.3. On the middle finger's central position, there is of course a general acknowledgement. However, if the thumb is kept aside, the remaining four fingers do not have a definite centre: the medial position is shared by the middle and the ring finger. Therefore, there are languages where the ring finger happens to be described as "the finger of the middle". One of these is Latin: cf. *medii digiti* (pl.) 'the middle fingers', with reference to the middle and the ring finger; more precisely, the ring finger is named *medius digitus minor* (ANDRÉ 1991: 102).

In Iranian, one may quote Krd. (Mukri) *qâmîk î nêwê* 'Mittel- und Ringfinger' (CHRISTENSEN – BARR 1939: 305). One could also explain in this light (Makrāni) Bal. *nyāmīen laŋkuk* 'ring finger' recorded by MORGENSTIERNE (1932a: 40), which otherwise should only be interpreted as a misunderstanding.[257] Even the usage of the term *gaḍḍī* ('middle finger') to name the ring finger, maintained by one of my Balochi (Mari) informants,[258] can be motivated by a sort of equation between middle and ring finger. But at this point, in order to avoid ambiguity, a specification is needed: the ring finger is the *kasānē gaḍḍī* ('the little *gaḍḍī*'), while, by contrast, the middle finger is the *mazanē gaḍḍī* ('the big *gaḍḍī*'). Similarly, the ring finger is described as a 'little middle finger' in Waxi and Rošani; cf. Wx. *mis:nam*

[256] The items recorded in ZARUBIN 1960 are morphologically plural (pl. suffix *-aθ*).

[257] Cf. FILIPPONE 2000–2003: 81 n. 70.

[258] None of the others, however, confirmed a similar use for *gaḍḍī*.

tsiklai (LORIMER 1958) and Roš. *khal-lakak* (SKÖLD 1936: 186), as contrasted respectively to *mis:na aŋgl* and *lakak iŋgax̌t* 'middle finger'. On Wx. *ʒəqlay* [*tsiklai*] and Roš. *khal* 'small' see below, pp. 152 f. and pp. 166 f.

4.1. If compared with the middle finger, the ring finger is certainly smalller. This comparison substantiates the existence of labels which depict this finger as a small(er) finger; cf. Wx. *zʌq/zǎq yʌngəl* (LORIMER 1958) with *zʌq* 'little, small', Yzɣ. *cəldůri ɣʷax̌t* with *cəldůr* 'smaller; younger', which is also a forefinger name (see above p. 130), and Pšt. *bačagúta, bačagwə́ta*, lit. the 'child [*bačá*] – finger'.

4.2. The ring finger names accounting for the finger dimension, however, mostly take the little finger as the touchstone. Such a comparison leads one to say that this finger is a 'bigger finger', as is illustrated by Gz. *engulī beleter* (ŽUKOVSKIJ 1922: 110), or a 'big little finger', as is illustrated by Yɣn. *kátta čīnčīlaq* or *kátta čīlīk* with *kátta* 'big' and *čīnčīlaq, čīlīk* 'little finger'. Should we interpret also Par. *aŋgušt-e bari* as a 'big finger', taking Par. *bari* (to my knowledge, otherwise unrecorded) as a lw. from IA (cf. CDIAL 11225 s.v. *vaḍra-* 'big')? However, this suggestion needs to be reinforced by further evidence.

Doubtfully, one may also associate here Pšt. *xamta gúta*, quoted by RAVERTY (1860 s.v. *gūta'h*) as an Eastern Pšt. name of the ring finger: *xamta* could perhaps be interpreted as the fem. form (*xamáṭa*) of *xamáṭ* 'plump, chubby; fat, stout'.

5. In WIr., and in particular Southern and Central Kurdish, Gorāni and Central dialects, the ring finger and the little finger are depicted as related each other by a kinship degree. To the ring finger, which is bigger and very close to the little finger, the protective function of an elder versus a younger sibling is attributed. It may perceived (1) as the little finger's brother, as proved by SulKrd. *bira y tûte*, SouthKrd. (*qâmkî*) *birâî tûta*(*l̲a*) (*angustî birâtûta* SAFIZĀDE 2001), Krmnš. *berâ tuta*, Gor. (Gahw.) *kilik-i berâ tûtä*, Gz. *engolī-birā-biländ* (lit. 'tall-brother-finger'), or (2) as the little finger's mother, as proved by Xur. *māyekelēč* (*māye kleič* FARAHVAŠI 1976), NBšk. (Sardašt) *mom-kukalü*, SBšk. (Garu) *makukalu* (G. BARBERA p.c.). Ring finger names based on kinship relations are found in other languages as well; the ring finger as the mother of the little finger is found, for example, in Celtic (POTT 1847: 295) and in Modern Uigur (*çimçılaq anası* lit. 'the mother of the little finger' ERDAL 1981: 124).

To a degree of kinship among fingers could also point KurmKrd. *babelîçk* (RIZGAR 1993; *bobeliçk* FARISOV 1957, (*tilyâ*) *bâbilîčk* AWRANG 1969, *tilyâ bâbilîçk* SAFIZĀDE 2001), as well as KurmKrd. *mamelisk* (KURDOEV 1960), SouthKrd. *mâmelînčk*, all meaning 'ring finger'. All of them could be analysed as derivatives from the Krd. address terms for 'father, daddy' (*bab, bav*) and 'paternal uncle' (*mâma*/*mame*). Note however that *babelîçk* (*bâblîčk*) is recorded as 'little finger' in HAŽĀR 1990 and SAFIZĀDE 2001, and as 'middle finger' in EBRĀHIMPUR 1994b (s.v. *angošt*).

6. A metaphorical association assuming the botanical world as the source domain has probably produced Pšt. *lākúlakáṛa* 'ring finger', which however has been recorded as 'middle finger' in Wanetsi (ELFENBEIN 1984).[259] The image evoked by this name is that of a straight, pointed finger, which for its shape is equated to a *lakáṛa* (< IA, cf. CDIAL 10875), i.e. a stick, a reed. As for *lāk°*, the initial part of the Pšt. idiom, should we think to a meaningless lexical element for an echo-copulative-compound?

7. Bohr. *eŋguš*, Voniš. *uŋguss*, Keš. *aŋguss* are general words for 'finger' used as names for the ring finger.

8. As far as Prs. *benser* 'ring finger' is concerned, one may only say that this is an Ar. loanword (cf. Ar. *binṣir*, Syr. *beṣrâ* in MAŠKUR 1978) with a very limited usage, being restricted to the scientific lexicon (MOINFAR 1981: 230). It is labelled as "rare" in LAZARD 1990a.

9. The following ring finger names have proved difficult to analyze: Taj. *angušt-i zinhor* (recorded as 'forefinger' in Prs. dictionaries);[260] Taj. (Kara-Tegin) *čabliki* (ROZENFEL'D 1982); Taj. *angušt-i (lelak-i) dastpūšak* (cf. dial. Taj. *dastpūša* 'glove' ROZENFEL'D 1982 ?); KurmKrd. *belîcan* (RIZGAR 1993).

---

259 Cf. above, p. 141.
260 Cf. above, p. 124.

CHAPTER SEVEN: THE LITTLE FINGER

1. The salient feature of the little finger which has mostly influenced naming processes in languages all over the world is its small size. A few examples of this natural, elementary pattern are in VEENKER 1981: 371–372. Many others could easily be added to them.

All the Iranian little finger names stress this physical characteristics, no special function being ascribed to this finger. However, smallness may be emphasized adopting alternative lexical strategies. It is possible, for example, to simply describe the finger as small, or "the small(est)", and in this case the various idioms differ as regards the specific terms for 'small' they contain. It is possible to grant to this finger the status of a child. Among all the fingers, it is the most natural to conceive as the youngest, the last born. The languages adopting a DIGIT = HUMAN BEING equation very frequently present the LITTLE FINGER = CHILD equation; for some instances see BROWN – WITKOSKI 1981: 602 (Table 4). But since most of the Iranian terms used in expressions for 'little finger' cover both the sense of 'small' and that of 'baby, small child', it is hardly ever possible to discriminate between the two different strategies. For this reason, the labels depicting the little finger as the small(est) finger or the young(est) "child-finger" are gathered together in §§ 1.1–15 below, grouped according to their etymological affiliation.

1.1. The standard Persian name of the little finger is *angošt-e kučak,* with *kučak* 'small, little, young', an adjective of very common usage, already documented in Middle Persian; cf. MPrs. *kūč(ak)* 'small'.

To Prs. *kučak* and *kučulu* 'small, tiny, little child, etc.', many similar Ir. forms are connected. Apart from colloquial Prs., Esf.Prs. *kučik* 'small', *kučuli*, *quzuli* 'tiny, minute', AfγPrs. (Kāb.) *kočak* (BAU 2003), Haz. *kej̆lʌk* 'short', etc., (sure or possible) cognates are found (1) in the whole Lori and Fārs area (Bxt. *kučir*, (ČLang) *kučik, kočir*, Lo. *koček*, (Bālā-Gar.) *kučik*, Šušt. *kočok*, Ban. *kuček̂*, Mosq., Rič., Baliā., Birov., Hay., Dāreng., Dežg. *kučik̂*, Gorgn. *koček̂*, Kal. (Lor) *kočok̂*, Nud., Pāp., Gorgn., Knd. *koŝkak̂*; Kāz., Mās. *kuŝkak̂*; Mamas. *koškolu*, Dašt., Dādenǰ. *kočik*, Buš. *kučil*, Dav. *xu:ǰak*; *xu:ǰmalek*); (2) in Central dialects (Gz. *kučūlī*, Anār. *kučču* (LECOQ 2002) 'small', Sirǰ. *kočku* 'very small', ZorYzd. *kūčīl*); (3) in Caspian and North-Iran dialects (Gil. *kuči*, *kučtə, kuštə, kuštay, kučə, kučik, kučikə*, Damāv. *kočik*, Māz. (Sār.) *kučik, kučinā, kučināk*, IrĀz. *kičik* (NAVĀBI 1992), (Sagz.) *qiǰil*, Tāl. *gaǰ*, IrĀz. *geč*

(ABDOLI 2001: 244)); (4) in the Kurdish and Zāzā areas (KurmKrd. *qicik* 'small, little', SouthKrd. *kučkok, kička, gučik, gičik, gičko, gička, gičkoka* 'small', *qičik, qîč, gičkoḻa, gičkaḻa* 'small, tiny', *qinǰik* 'a little', *xuǰok* 'very small'), Zā. (Šeyxān) *qiž,* (Kulp) *qiǰ,* (Varto) *qičkēk* 'small, young', (Çermik) *qeček* 'child' (see also HADANK 1932: 296). Note also Prs. *kič* 'small, tiny', *kič-kič* 'scattered' (a dial. term?). Connected forms are found in EIr. as well; cf. Pšt. *kučnáy* 'small; little', *kučóṭay, kəčóṭay* 'tiny, small', Oss. *gyccyl,* (Dig.) *giccil* 'small'.

As far as the names of the little finger are concerned, besides Prs. *angošt-e kučak*, one may quote Šir. *kelenǰe kučike* (XADIŠ 2000), Mās. *penǰe-y kočku*, Birov. *penǰe-y kučeku,* Hay., Dādenǰ., Rič. *penǰe-y kučku*, Mamas. *k̂e-lič-e košku*, Kal. (Tāǰ.), Nud., Pāp., Mosq., Kal. (Lor) *penǰe-y košku*, Dāreng. *penǰe-y kučik̂*, Dežg. *penǰe-y kučeku*, Ban. *penǰe-y kuček*, SouthKrd. *qala kučk*, Zā. *engişta qij* (TODD 1985), Bxt. *keliče* (*angošt*) *kučire* (my own data), Gil. *kuči angušt(əy)* (PĀYANDE 1987, s.v. *angoštān-e dast*), *kučələ an-gušt* (SOTUDE 1963), Qasr. *angušd kučikak*, Sed. *uŋgulī-kičī/kučulī*, Buš. *kičul*(*uk*), Lir.-Dayl. *kičul* (LIRĀVI 2001: 272), Dašt. *kičluk, kičiluk, kilčuk*, ZorYzd. *angušt-i kūčūlōg*, Gz. *ə̆ŋgolī-kučulī,* and in EIr., Pšt. *kə́ča gúta/ gwə́ta, xáča gúta, xačə́y gúta, xačə́y mačə́y gúta* (also *kīča gúta* in RAVERTY 1860 s.v. *gūta'h*), *kučnáy gwə́ta, kačəy gwə́ta* (QALANDAR MOMAND – SHE-RAYI 1994), Wan. *xəčəkangut,* (ELFENBEIN 1984) *xəčə́y mučə́y* and Dzadr. *xčə́nkye*.

Pšt. *xačə́y mačə́y gúta* and Wan. *xəčə́y mučə́y* are instances of the Ir. echo-compound, or alliterative compound type, where the second element is devoid of meaning and repeat approximately the first element with the change of its first consonant (generally with an *m*-sound), as is the case with Prs. *baččе-mačče* 'a mere boy' (STEINGASS 1963), also used as a pragmatically marked reference to a plurality of children. Other instances are mentioned above and below in this book (see e.g. Bal. *čūncī mačūnčī* 'little finger', § 5 below). Pšt. *xačə́y mačə́y gúta* might help understand Pšt. *xamə́ča gúta* 'little finger'. According to RAVERTY 1860, Pšt. *xamə́ča* means 'puny, petty, short', but this word seems to be only used in collocation with words for 'finger' and 'rib' in lexicalized phrases meaning 'little finger' and 'short ribs' (*xamə́ča puxtə́y*). My suggestion is considering *xamə́ča* as a 'contracted' form of an echo-compound, based on *xáča* 'small'.[261]

---

[261] ASLANOV (1966) does not provide a Russian equivalent of *xamə́ča*; he quotes (s.v.) the two lexicalized phrases containing *xamə́ča* which have been mentioned above.

1.2. Prs. *kučak* and cognates have been connected to an Ir. base **kau-/ku-* 'young, small', which may be envisaged in several words for 'small' in Prs. and other Ir. languages, and explained as < **kau-ča-ka-* (literature in SZEMERÉNYI 1977: 15). There is a more or less general agreement on this derivation, and there is no reason to challenge it. However, I would like to stress that the syllabic structure of Prs. *kučak* goes perfectly well with the sound symbolic patterns evocative of the concept of SMALLNESS, we find in other words for 'small', as can be easily verified looking at many of the terms gathered in the following paragraphs.[262] Sound symbolism is a much productive, not-arbitrary naming process which links associations of vowels and consonants with the human perception of size, shape, material consistency, movement, sound (onomatopoeia), etc.[263] It may also provide a good explanation for the very large lexical cluster to which Bal. *čuk* 'child' belongs. Discussing Khot. *cakvaka-* 'boy', MAGGI (1997a: 64–67 and 1997b) quotes Bal. *čuk* and some relevant items (in EIr. and WIr., IA and Dravidian), which present a "similarity" with the Khot. term. MAGGI's list could easily be enlarged: cf. e.g. Haz. *čvqʌj, čvqnʌj* 'small, little', AfγPrs. *čukāčukī, čukāpukī* 'a little' (ŠĀLČI 1991), Sist. *čok, čokak* 'a little' and many others. In Krd., besides the *čuk/čûk* forms quoted by MAGGI, *čik*-forms are also found: cf. e.g. SouthKrd. *čik, čikê* 'a little'. A nasal insertion seems also possible: cf. AfγPrs. *čungī* 'small' (ŠĀLČI 1991), which reminds Bal. *čunkī* 'little finger' (see below). MAGGI, who also quotes a few examples in languages other than Iranian, like e.g. It. *cucciolo*, states that «their similarity, and on the other hand, [...] the general lack of precise phonological correspondences» would lead «to the conclusion that the words under consideration are onomatopoeic formations that have arisen and evolved independently, at least in part, in the various languages» (1997a: 66).[264] However, while it is certainly true that the iconicity based on sound symbolism often

---

262 Note that ABAEV (IESOJ) explains Oss. *gyccyl* 'small' as belonging to child language («s "detskim" slovom»).

263 An interdisciplinary collection of studies on this much productive device is HINTON – NICHOLS – OHALA 1994. A comprehensive examination of how it affects the Iranian lexicon is still a desideratum. At a first sight, it seems reasonable to state that affricate segments (palato-alveolar [tʃ] – [dʒ] and also alveo-dental [ts] –[dz] in EIr., possibly preceded or followed by high frequency vowels) may concur to evoke SMALLNESS, being frequently found in words meaning 'small' and/or 'child' and/or 'small of animals'.

264 Though admitting a relationship between Khot. *cäkvaka-* and Wx. *cuk* 'small', TREMBLAY (2000: 193) prefers envisaging a popular borrowing from an Indian language, on account of the direct resemblance of the Khot. word with Skt. *cikva-* 'baby elephant'.

appears to have a universal character, I still think that the prevalence of specific sound patterns as contrasted with other possible ones in a given linguistic area (as large as may be, and irrespective of the localization of an irradiation centre) may be recognized as a shared areal feature.

Derivatives from *čuk* ‘child’ occur in the following Bal. idioms: *čukī lankuk* (mainly SBal.: Karachi, Dašt, Kasarkand), *čukkī čangul* (Irānšahr), *čukkol* (Sarāwān), *čunkī* (Turbat) ‘little finger’. To them, KurmKrd. *t’ilîya ç’ûk* ‘pinkie, little finger’ is connected.

Yzγ. *cəgagi γ^{w}ax̌t* ‘little finger’ contains *cəgag* ‘small, little’. According to SKÖLD (1936: 186), both *ts^{ə}gagi u̯ax̌t* and (with comparative) *tsəgagtar u̯ax̌t* ‘small finger’ are in use. Wx. *zʌqi̇q yəŋgəl* ‘little finger’ (LORIMER 1958) contrasts with *zʌq yʌngəl* ‘ring finger’ (lit. ‘the small finger’),[265] in that it describes the former as smaller than the latter (Wx. *zʌqi̇q* ‘little, small, smaller than *zʌq*’). In fact, it is always possible to make graded assessments in measure evaluation.

As *l*-extensions of bases that could be linked to Bal. *čuk*, all meaning ‘small, little’, ‘child’ or the like, the following may be considered: SouthKrd. *čikol̲a, čikala, čikol̲uka, čikoloka*, etc. ‘small’, *čikolâna* ‘very small’, Mahâb. *čikōla* ‘small’, Šušt. *ǰeqele* ‘little child’ (FĀZELI 2004), Bxt. (ČLang) *ǰeqela*, (Pāgač) *ǰeqele* ‘boy’, IrĀz. (Ebr.) *ǰeqel*, (Čā.) *zeqela* ‘small’, Gil. *ǰaɣal*, *ǰeqel* ‘baby, small child’ (*ǰaqalə* PĀYANDE 1987, s.v. *bačče* and *čakâl* ‘small, tiny’ SOTUDE 1963), (Māč.) *ǰaγ^{ə}l* ‘child’, Damāv. (echo-compound) *ǰeqel beqel* ‘(many) small children’, Tāl. *ǰək(ə)la* (*čoxla* in Astar), Xor. (Mašhad) *ǰeqeli* ‘small (i.e. having small limbs, of human beings); small child’ (ADIB TUSI 1963–1964), TrbHayd. *ǰeqeli* ‘small’ and *zoqula* ‘small child’, Zand (Tafreš area) *ǰiqil* (MOQDAM 1949: 27), Qm. *zeqele* ‘small child’, Esf.Prs. *ǰeγele* ‘a little man’, Buš. *ǰeγele* ‘boy’, Lārest. *čikala* ‘chick; nestling’ (ADIB TUSI 1963–1964), Farām. *čikal(u)* ‘chick’, etc. These terms outline a compact band stretching from West Iran (Kurdish and Baxtiāri areas), and North Iran up to Xorāsān, but similar forms are also in use along the Southern Iranian belt. Possibly, a Sgd. antedecent is recorded in the Prs.-Sgd. glossary fragment M 425, where in V/3, in connection with Man. MPrs. *qwdk* (*kōdak* ‘small’), the Sgd. characters <cγ’> is readable. MORANO (2005: 219–220) suggests emending it as *cγ’[lyẖ]*, and his suggestion seems quite convincing.

As little finger names, one may quote Mukri *qâmîk î čkôlah* (CHRISTENSEN – BARR 1939: 305) and Gil. *čakale angušt*, with the metathesized variant *čalake-angušt*. Similarly, in EIr. we find Wx. *ʒəqlay yangląk* ‘little

[265] See above, p. 147.

finger' from *ʒəqlay, cəqlay* 'small, little'.[266] According to LORIMER 1958, Wx. *tsiklai* is both 'finger' and 'little finger'.

1.3. It is not clear whether KurmKrd. *piç'ûk, biç'ûk* 'small, little; child' is connected to Prs. *bačče* 'child' and its several cognates. As for Krd., CABOLOV 2001 points to an older **čû-* 'small'. He suggests separating the Krd. word from the *bačče*-lexical set, for which in IESOJ (s.v. *biccew* 'child') an etymology based on a common Ir., Caucasian, IA substratum is proposed.

The situation is much entangled and CABOLOV's explanation appears unconvincing. For Kurdish one may quote KurmKrd. *buçuk, biçuk, biçîk, biç'ûk, biç'ûçik, piç'ûk* 'small; child', *piçek, bîç'ek* 'a little', Sul. *pich* 'small quantity', *pichûk, bichûk* 'little, small', *beç* 'young, child', SouthKrd. *bučk, bučka, bička, bičuk, bičûk, pičuk, bičučk, bičkok, bičola, pičkoḻ, bičkol,* etc. 'small', *bučân, bučkalâna, bičkalâna, bičkolâna, bičkaḻa, pičkala* 'very small', *pêčika* 'a newborn baby', Krmnš. *beč* 'any small thing'. To these Krd. forms, add Zā. *pičēke* 'a little', Gor. (Talahed.) *büček* 'small', Māz. (Āmol.) *pečik* 'very small', Ardest. *pači* 'a little', Dav. *peča* 'a little; a tiny fragment; a small quantity of a thing', Kor. *biček* 'small', Lārest. *peči* 'a little' (ADIB TUSI 1963–1964) and many others, among which Šušt. *bačila* and Buš. *bočil* 'chick'. See also (Gypsy) Zand *büčok* 'small' (MOQDAM 1949: 80). An isolated, connected form is found in the Tajik dialect of the Kulyāb valley; cf. *piči* 'a little' in ROZENFEL'D 1982. I would also include in this set the word *pyš* 'a little' occurring in a Geniza fragment written with Hebrew characters in an Iranian dialect, probably Northern or Central (SHAKED 1988: 225).

Krd. forms belonging to the *piç'ûk/ pičuk* set occur in the following names of the little finger: KurmKrd. *telîya pečûk* (*tilîya biçuk*), SulKrd. *emusty pichûk,* Kor. *kelek-e biček*, Gor. (Talahed.) *kelek büčkala.* In Sivandi, *pīčeke* 'little finger' has been recorded by ANDREAS and quoted by EILERS 1988 and LECOQ 1979.[267]

As for EIr., I would quote here Baǰ. *bicik ingaxt*, with Baǰ. *bicik* connected to Roš. and Xuf. *buc* (m.), *bic* (f.) 'baby, small child', etc. Differently, MORGENSTIERNE (EVŠG) relates Šγn., Xuf., Roš., Baǰ., Oroš. *-buc* (m.), *-bic* (f.) 'child, young (of animal)' to Šγn., Xuf., Roš., Baǰ., Oroš. *puc*, Yzγ. *poc* etc. 'son', and consequently to Av. *puθra-*. May we think here of a contamination between forms with different etymologies? In fact, Ir. **θr* > Šγn.

---

[266] See also STEBLIN-KAMENSKIJ 1999 s.v.

[267] LECOQ lists it among the words appeared in previous publications, which have not been confirmed by his informants (1979: 200).

c does not account for all Šγn. *c*. Throughout EVŠG, the cases of Šγn. *c-* / *-c-* / *-c* < **θr*, which may be considered as sure, i.e. substantiated by attestations in other Ir. languages, as is case with *puc* 'son', *pōc* 'time', *yōc* 'fire', and not hypothesized, often with many doubts by MORGENSTIERNE himself, are very few. The other cases are mostly well explained with the fact that Šγn. *c* often corresponds to *č* in other Ir. languages. In my view, MORGENSTIERNE's statement as regards *ceg* 'child, suckling', that «If genuine ŠGr-Y word *c-* < * *θr-*, but poss. a migratory word, cf. CDIAL 4781 s.v. *cikka*³-» is open to question.[268] One should probably not think that all the Šuγni words starting with *c-*, which cannot be derived from **θr-* (like for example Šγn. *cōm* 'eye'), have to be considered as not "genuine" Šuγni words.

1.4 Tāl. *munǰilə, munǰlə, mužlə, muǰil, mu(n)ǰilə angĭštə* 'little finger' may be hardly separated from Tāl. *miǰa* 'small', which ABDOLI (2001: 171) ascribes to child language.

Mnǰ. *mlemčigha* 'little finger' is in some way reminiscent of Tāl. *munǰilə*; if the two forms are actually related is doubtful.

To Tāl. *miǰa* 'small' are connected Māz. (Āmol.) *mičkak* 'very small', Dav. *mu:ǰak* 'small; having small limbs', and probably also Yγn. *muččonak, muččunak* 'small' (MIRZOZODA 2008).

1.5. Ār.-Bidg. *əgüšvêǰiǰ*, Bohr. *eŋgüst vüǰija*, Abiā. *angöšta vüǰüčče* 'little finger' contain an adjectival base for 'small' with several cognates in Central dialects. They are Vfs. *viǰa, viǰila* (MOQDAM 1949), *vílǰæ* (STILO 2004), Qm. *vezele*, Biz. *veǰīǰ* (*veǰiǰä* in MAZRAᶜTI *et al.* 1995), Ār.-Bidg. *vêǰiǰ*, Abiā. *vüǰüč*, Qohr. *vüǰǰa* (also 'cadet'), *vüǰüǰ*, Jawš. *vučul*, Mei. *vi:šli*, Vaǰguni *vi:šl, vi:šla* (SHAKIBI GUILANI – QOLIZADE VAZVANI 1990), Mah. (Vārān) *višl* (MAJIDI 1975: 63), etc. all meaning 'small'.

1.6. Siv. *gusse čilū* (ŽUKOVSKIJ 1922: 110) 'little finger' is a lexicalized phrase containing the adjective *čilū* 'small'; cf. also Siv. *čilkunū, čilekunū, čilukunū, čilikunū* 'very young, young(-er/est)', «an ‚absoluter Komparativ'» (EILERS 1988). According to EILERS, Siv. *čil-* is a «Kürzung (..) aus (np.) *kū-čilū*». I disagree with this explanation. By the way, it is worth noting that the ending *-(u)nū*, intensifying in this word the notion of SMALLNESS or imply-

---

[268] See also above p. 151 and fn. 263.

ing a comparison in the evaluation, is also found in Lārestāni; cf. Lārest. *kaidenû* 'smaller', from *kaidû* 'small, little', for which see below p. 161.

Siv. *čilū* has counterparts both in WIr. and EIr. In WIr., one may cite Semn. *čili čili* 'very small', Māz. *čelik* 'baby; little, young; small' (Sār. *čilik*, AliĀb. *čelik*), IrĀz. (ADIB TUSI 1992: no. 1180) *čelik* 'small', *čelêin* 'newborn baby; small and fragile', Tāl. *čilaza* 'child, infant' (ABDOLI 2001), Damāv. *čelka,* KurmKrd. *çelîk* 'young of bird' (RIZGAR 1993 *çêlik̠* 'young animal [kitten, puppy, chick etc.]'), SouthKrd. *čêla* 'child', Zā. *čēlīk* 'young animal', Dašt. *čel zan* 'little woman', *čel merd* 'little man', Bast. *čilāki* '(small) chick', Her. *čel mardak* 'very short man' etc. In EIr., cognates to Siv. *čilū* are mostly found in the Šuγni group: cf. Šγn. *ʒul, ʒulik(ik),* fem. *ʒal, ʒalik(ik)* 'small; little, young', Sariq. *ʒïl, ʒůl* etc.[269]

Siv. *gusse čilū* may be compared with Biz. *čelīk*, perhaps also IrĀz. *ǰuli* (ADIB TUSI 1963–1964), Šγn. *ʒalik(ik) angix̌t* (ZARUBIN 1960), Sariq. *ʒïlag-ïngax̌t, ʒůlaq-ingax̌t*, Yzγ. *cəlyagī* (GAUTHIOT 1916), all meaning 'little finger'.

It could also be possible that the words for 'finger', such as Taj. *čilik*, which have been treated above, p. 65 and for which a connection to words for twigs, pieces of wood etc., has been suggested, would in fact belong here.

1.5. Prs. lexicographers record many expressions for 'little finger', some of which are not in use anymore, or have dialectal or other specific connotations. In any case, they are not in use in Standard Persian of Iran. Among these, there is *angošt-e xord(ak)*, *angošt-e xordin*, *xord angošt* (DEHX), to which one may link Taj. *angušt-i xurd* (also *čilik-i-xurd(i)* KALBĀSI 1995, *panǰa-i xurda* MIRZOZODA 2008, s.v. *naxna*), Šahm. *xord-engošt,* Abd. *penǰe-y xordek̂* (*xurdeḱ* in ŽUKOVSKIJ 1922: 110), Dorun. *penǰe-y xork̂ak̂*, Somγ. *penǰe-y xordu*, Ir.Bal. (Irānšahr) *urdūkē angušt* 'little finger'.

Prs. *xord* (superl. *xordin*) is recorded in dictionaries as 'small, minute; young; broken to pieces; change (money)'; its derivative *xorde* means 'bit, fragment; anything small; dust etc.'. Variants in informal registers are *xurd* and *xurde*; to colloquial Persian also belongs *xert*, which is only found in idioms like *xert-o-pert*, *xert-o-xurt* (NAJAFI 1999) 'trumpery'. For Eastern Persian, one may quote AfγPrs. *xərd* 'small; young' (BAU 2003), Xor. *xurd* 'small; a little', Madagl. *xerd* 'small', *xerdūna* 'kid', *xertīk* 'small, little',

[269] In EVŠG, s.v. (Yzγ.) *cəl-dûr* 'younger', MORGENSTIERNE doubtfully suggests a connection with the IA words assembled in CDIAL 4911; see also CDIAL 4877. I think there are good reasons to speak of an areal lexical family even in this case.

Sist. *xurd* 'small', *xurda* 'dust taken from the tomb of a saint, which, rubbed on body or eaten, is used as a remedy against illness; kid and lambs; change (of money)'. The *xord*-type adjectives have a large diffusion in Fārs, as well; cf. Dav. *xord, xordek, xordelek*, Dahl., Abd. *xordek̂*, Kāz., Kuz. *xord*, etc. (SALĀMI 2004: 174–177, s.vv. *kučak* and *riz*), Pāp. *xord* 'tiny', Somγ. *xord* 'small' (SALĀMI 2005: 176–178, s.vv. *kučak* and *riz*), Dorun. *xork̂ak̂* 'small' (SALĀMI 2006: 189, s.v. *kučak*), etc.

Prs. *xord* and *xorde* directly continue Phl. *xwurd* 'small, little, minute; of no value' and *xwurdag* 'something small; particle; detail', both unrecorded in Man. MPrs. Cognates to Prs. *xord* and *xorde* are numberless all over WIr. and EIr. and are also found as loanwords in Armenian and Caucasian languages (GIPPERT 2009). They differ as to the meaning they convey and their status inside the lexicon of the relevant languages. In some varieties, *xord*-forms are used as current adjectives for 'small', with a dimensional value, sometimes conveying the sense of 'child' or 'small domestic animal'; in some other varieties they are not so commonly used, having the restricted sense of 'minute, tiny; crushed', or being used as nominals to denote different kinds of very small and/or insignificant things.

In WIr., cognates to Prs. *xord* are KurmKrd. *xort* 'young; young man, youth', *hûr* 'small, petty (change); tiny, fine, minute', *xirt* 'three-year-old ram, male sheep', SorKrd. *wurd* 'small (esp. of children under ten years old); precise, attentive', SouthKrd. *xurd, urd, urt, ur, hur* 'small, minute; orderly and intelligent person', *xirt* 'trumpery', *wird* 'small, tiny', *wirda* 'lambs and kids; trumpery; a little bit', etc., Gor. (Kand.) *wird, wirdä* 'in pieces, crumbled', *wirdîklä* 'child', (Awr.) *wᴜrd* 'small, fine', Zā. *werdī* 'small' (Çermik-Siverek dial. area; PAUL 1998: 212), (Kur) *hôrdi, wurdi* 'small, in pieces', (Bij.) *wärdi* 'small', Bxt. (ČLang) *xird, hird* 'small', Lak. *hirdaru* 'small; generally, the smallest child in a family', Lo. *hird* 'small, minute', *hirdela* 'very small', *hirderu* 'all the children of a family'.

In North and Central Iran one finds IrĀz. (Ker.) *herden* 'child, baby', Tāl. *xerdan*, IrĀz. *xerde*, (Langarāni) *hrdan* 'baby' (ABDOLI 2001: 184–185), Šahm. *xord, xordenak* 'small', Sang. *xwrd* 'small', *xɛrtɛ* 'small' (AZAMI – WINDFUHR 1972), Māz. (Sār.) *xurd*, Qasr. *xurda* 'small' (DEYHIM 2005: 31), Vfs. *hurd* "small, tiny, broken up", Kah. *xurde*, Jawš. *hyrd* 'small', Abiā. *hǖrd* 'crumb', *ǖrda* 'a little', Biz. *xōrd* 'small, tiny', *xūrda* 'small, tiny; a little', Anār. *xurde* 'small' (LECOQ 2002), Nāi. *xird* 'small, tiny', *xirde* 'in pieces' (LECOQ 2002), Qohr. *hǖr*, Tār. *hürt*, Varz. *hirde* 'small, tiny', Del. *xeurd, xeud* 'small, little', Xuns. *hĭrt* '(short and) small' (EILERS 1976), Siv. *ferd* 'small', etc.

Cognates to Prs. *xord* are also found in Balochi: cf. WBal. *hūrt, hūrd, xūrt, (h)urta(g)* 'crushed, ground; small, tiny; small domestic animals', *hūrdag* 'material taken form a Pir's tomb and rubbed on body, or eaten etc. as a protection against evil'[270] (ELFENBEIN 1990-II), SBal. *(h)īrt, īrdag* (also *hūrt*) 'small, delicate; thin; fine, powdery; crumbs, powder, pieces; kids and lambs' (SAYAD HASHMI 2000), EBal *hīrθ* 'thin, fine; small', *hīrθen whaškī* 'small game' (MAYER 1909:171), etc. Bal. speakers from different areas of Iran tend to use *(h)urd*, *(h)urt*, *(h)urdūk* (my own data; *hord* 'small, young' in AYYUBI 2002) as an usual word for 'small' in many senses, in collocation with words denoting any kinds of referents having smaller dimensions as compared with other objects of the same category (such as mountains, trees, chairs, books, noses, human beings, etc.).

Among the small things which may be denominated with *xord*-type words, there are the small bones (Prs. *xorde ostoxān* [LAZARD 1990a, ĀRYĀNPUR KĀŠĀNI 1979] 'group of small bones'), in particular those composing hands and feet (Prs. *xord(e-ye) dast* 'wrist', *xorde ostoxān-e dast* 'carpus'; *xorde ostoxān-e pā* 'tarsus', Sang. *xūrdœ* 'knuckles' AZAMI – WINDFUHR 1972, SouthKrd. *xirtka, xirtik* 'joints of hands and feet'), or those of the ankle (Dav. *xordakun* 'malleolus', Prs. *xord-gāh* 'pastern of a quadruped', SulKrd. *xirtke, xirke* 'ankle-joint, pastern-joint'). A Bal. speaker from Noške, gave me *ūrtband* as 'knuckle-joints'; he was probably influenced by Brahui, his mother tongue (cf. Br. *xūrt band* 'wrist, ankle' < Ir., but from which language?; ROSSI 1979: F100). The oldest attestation of this usage is in Phl.; cf. *xwurdag* '(horse's) pastern', e.g. in *GrBd.* 24.13.

To the *xord*-group belongs Par. *γuṛṑk*[271] 'child' according to MORGENSTIERNE (IIFL-I: 257, EVP: 92 Par. *γuṛṑk* < **wr̥ta-*: Prs. *xurd* < **hwr̥ta-*), who also suggests connecting here Pšt. *woṛ, wuṛ, wəṛ* 'small; tiny; short; insignificant' (EVP s.v. *wuṛ, wōṛ*, but more cautiously in NEVP < ***wr̥ta*-?). TREMBLAY (2005: 183) has contested this connection, but his derivation of the Pšt. word (< **baratá-* 'dont il faut s'occuper', with an early syncopation of the middle vowel) seems unconvincing, at least from the semantic/conceptual point of view.

---

270 There is no reason to resort to «NP *xwar-*», as in ELFENBEIN 1990-II; the material which is rubbed on the body is 'earth, dust', i.e. a thing with a fair chance of being named "the pulverised". I take the opportunity to remark that the possible direct origin of Br. *xuṛda, xwaṛda* 'dust taken from the shrine of a saint' and *xūrda* 'lamb' is Sistāni (cf. ROSSI 1979: H 741, H743).

271 According to KIEFFER, Par. *γ(o)ṛók, γ(o)ṛṑk* 'enfant' is a word well understood, but never used spontaneously, by his Par. informants (1979: 261).

On the etymology of Prs. *xord* and its numberless cognates all over WIr. and (possibly) EIr., no agreement has been reached. Among the hypotheses advanced so far, one may quote that in Horn 1893 (√*qert-* 'schneiden', suggested by Nöldeke but contested by Hübschmann 1895: 57); Morgenstierne 1937: 347 (< **hw-r̥ta-* 'well-ground'); Nyberg 1931: 134 («*t*-Erweiterung zu *χōr*» 'deep'); Eilers 1957: 335 (< PIr. **x*^{w}*ar-* 'to eat, to consume'); Cipriano 1998: 252 (< Av. *x*^{v}*ara-* 'wound, sore', < IE **swVr-* 'to wound', already in de Lagarde, disputed by Horn), where a semantic connection with Prs. *x*^{w}*ār* 'despised, wretched' is envisaged. Eilers' "eaten"-hypothesis is old; it had already been basketed by Horn, in view of the *u*-vocalism of the MPrs. form (as contrasted to the "regular" *xwa°* of *xwardan* 'to eat'). Recently, Gippert (2009: 137–138) has resumed this etymology, reconstructing a form **xwr̥ta-*, which «may well represent the original past participle "eaten" of the root **xwar-*». As a support to this derivation, he mentions semantic parallels from Germanic (Engl. *bit*, Germ. *Bisschen*, from a verb meaning 'to bite').

In my view, however, many *xord*-cognates cannot be explained on the basis of Gippert's suggestion, though it is always possible to think to lexical contamination and overlapping, with the subsequent alteration of the expected phonetic changes, and I still consider Morgenstierne's etymology as more reliable. The PULVERISED, CRUSHED → SMALL conceptual derivation represents an iconomastic type: see for instance Khot. *ñaḍa-* 'small' (if < **ni-arta-* 'ground down', as in Bailey 1979; 22, 116), Skt. *kṣudrá-* 'small, tiny' (EWA I: 434, CDIAL 3712) and a few other semantic parallels in Buck 1949: 880-881. One could also add here Taj. *mayda*, for which see below, § 1.14.

In his attempt to explain Badaxš. *xetārik* 'small, little', which occurs in the lexicalized phrase *lakük/likīk i xetārik* 'little finger', Lorimer (1922: 178) points to a doubtful derivation from an attested *xertārik*, having probably Prs. *xord,* Madagl. *xerd* 'small', *xertīk* 'small, little' in mind. At present no final words can be said on the matter.

1.6. Prs. *angošt-e keh* and *angošt-e kehin(e)* 'little finger' contain *keh* and *kehin,* respectiveley the old comparative and superlative forms from an adjectival base not attested as such in Persian. We find it in Avestan (YAv. *kasu-* 'small, little'), in Sogdian (*kəs, kas* <'ks-, ks-> 'thin'), in Bactrian (*κασοκο, κοσοκο* 'little, a little, slightly', < **kasu-ka-* Sims-Williams 2000), in Man. Parthian (*kasišt* <qsyšt, ksyšt>), as far as old Ir. languages are concerned. As for MPrs., the Phl. writing <ks, ksyst> hides the actual pronunciation. Taking into account the Man. MPrs. spelling <kyh, qyh> and following the lines of MACKENZIE's transcription, I will conventionally quote the Phl. word as *keh* 'small(er), less(er), young(er)' (and *kehist* 'smallest'), exactly as I have done with Phl. <ms, msyst> (see above, p. 96).

Apart form Prs. *keh*, reflexes in Modern Iranian of Ir. **kasu-* are numerous and mainly spread in Central dialects, dialects of North and Caspian area, in Balochi and in a few EIr. languages. See Anār. *kas*, Ardest. *kēs, kēs(s)u*, Nāi. *kas*, Tār. *kas*, Varz. *kas*, Xur. *kēsu*, ZorYzd. *kas, kasūg, kasōg*, Yzd-JPrs. *kasok*, Keš. *kas*, Zefr. *kas*, Āšt. *kastar, kassar*, Āmor. *küsdarak*, Vonuš. *kessar*, Xuns. *kissar*, Ham-JPrs. *käsär*, Hanǰ. *kasla*, Sang., Semn., Lāsg., *kasin*, Srx. *kesin*, all meaning 'small', Sang. *kasinu* 'smaller' (*kas* in AZAMI – WINDFUHR 1972), etc.[272] See also Bal. *kasān* 'small' and, for EIr., Pšt. *kəšr, kə́šər, kíšər*, Oss. *k'äst'är* 'younger; cadet'.

That Av. (gen.) *kasištahe ərəzvō* (BARTHOLOMAE 1904 'des kleinesten Fingers'), with the corresponding Phl. expression *kehist angust* (*Vd.* 6.10) could be taken as the name of the little finger, has been suggested above, p. 96. In the Phl. documentation, one also finds *keh angust* 'little finger/toe' in *GrBd.* VII.10[273] and *WZ* 22.9 (*angust-ē homānāg keh* "comme un doigt, le plus petit", GIGNOUX – TAFAZZOLI 1993). Here also belong Aft. *kasin engošt*, Semn. *kasin angošt(a)*, Sang. *kas angoštu*, Tāl. (Kargānrudi) *gəsa angəšta* (D. GUIZZO p.c.), Zefr. *üŋgülī ḱasa,* Nat. *eŋgulī ḱas*, Gz. *ĕngolī-käs(e)*, ZorYzd. *angušt-i kasōg*, Bal. *kasānẽ lankuk* (Karachi and Nal)[274] and *kastarẽ lankuk* (from a Bal. speaker living in Oman), Oss. *kæstær ængwylʒ* (my own data) or *kæstær k'ūx*.

MORGENSTIERNE quotes (dial.) Pšt. *kašnəi gwəta* 'little finger' in EVP, s.v. *kašr*. Due to a misinterpretation of the abbreviation 'B' in EVP (= Twayer Khan from Bangash), which does not refer to a Bal. but to a Pšt. informant, PSTRUSIŃSKA (1974: 170 and 1985–1986, where *kasnəi:* is a misprint) mentions a non-existent Bal. *kašnəi gūta* 'little finger'. PSTRUSIŃSKA (1974: 169) underlines that Pšt. *kə́šər* 'younger' and *məšər* 'older' may only be used with reference to human beings. This means that, if Pšt. *kašnəi* in *kašnəi gwəta* is actually related to Pšt. *kə́šər*, this thumb name should be considered as a figurative expression. However, it is by no means certain that Pšt. *kašnəi* and *kə́šər* do have some relationship. The former is not mentioned in NEVP, nor in other etymological repertoires (see DE CHIARA 2008: 495). An alternative hypothesis, kindly suggested to me by M. DE CHIARA,

272 See also STILO 2007: 96 (and Table 2).

273 In this passage, *keh angust* is actually 'little toe' (since at the death of Gayōmard, the Evil Spirit first touches the little toe of his right leg).

274 On Bal. *kasānen* [*laŋkuk*] 'forefinger' (MORGENSTIERNE 1932a: 40) see above, p. 131.

is considering Pšt. *kašnəi* as a dialectal variant of Pšt. *kučnáy* 'small', for which see above, § 1.1.

1.7. The Khot. label for 'little finger', *kaṇaiska*, is in some way related to Skt. *kaniṣṭhā-* 'id.', fem. of *kaniṣṭhá-* '(RV) youngest, (Lex.) younger brother' (CDIAL 2718, 2719, with modern IA outcomes). To it, one may add Skt. (Lex.) *kanyasā-* and (Lex.) *kanīnī-, kanī́nakā-, kanī́nikā-* 'little finger' (fem. of respectively *kanyasa-* 'younger' and *kanīna-* 'young, youthful' (CDIAL 2735, 2736); see also EWA I: 297–298.

Khot. *kaṇaiska* 'little finger' is homophonous with the Khot. name of the famous Kushan king, Kanishka. Scholars have long since referred both to the Ir. base **kan-* (IE **ken-* 'to come forth freshly', IEW 1959: 563–564), from which words linked to the notion of YOUTH / SMALLNESS have developed; see BAILEY 1945: 21–22. The name of the king has been interpreted as the 'most youthful in vigour' by BAILEY 1954: 146. According to HENNING (1965: 82–84), should be analysed as **kaništa-ka-*, a Bactr. *-ka*-derivative from a superlative degree. EILERS 1970 pointed at an Ir. *-št-* > *-šk-* development. Taking into account the dental *-s-*, EMMERICK (1993: 53) challenged the assumed 'superlative' nature of this word: «*kaṇaiska* "little finger" cannot derive from **kaništa-ka-* (comparing **kaništa-* with the Old Indian superlative *kaniṣṭhá-*) because **šta-ka-* would almost certainly have resulted in *-ṣka-* in Khotanese». For EMMERICK, therefore, the Khot. name of the little finger may only be explained assuming an original **kaniča-ka-* > **kaniska-*, which subsequently «was blended with **kaṇaiṣka-* < Bactrian *κανηþκο* with the consequence that both resulted in *kaṇaiska-* in Khotanese». While EMMERICK's position is well founded on the phonological level, the semantic arguments he adduces in support of his analysis («There is of course no reason why the "little finger" (Modern Persian *angošt-e kuček*) need be named as the "littlest"») may be questioned on account, at least, of Skt. *kaniṣṭhā-* 'little finger'.

In many Ir. languages, the Ir. base **kan-* has developed derivative nouns with the specialized sense of 'girl'; cf. Prs. *kaniz* 'girl, female slave' and its several cognates. Outcomes of **kan-* have been collected in etymological dictionaries; see BAILEY 1979, s.v. *kaṇaiska* and IESOJ, s.v. *k'annəg*. As belonging to **kan-*, with a semantic range going from 'small' (in many senses) to 'short', besides Oss. *k'annəg* 'small', I would quote KurmKrd. *kin* 'short (of stature)',[275] possibly Sang. *qɛnar* 'small' (AZAMI – WINDFUHR 1972) and

[275] So also CHYET 2003, quoting CABOLOV 1976: 11; a different understanding is in CABOLOV 2001 s.v. [< *OIr. *kuntaka-*]).

Farām. *kengel*, Bast. *kengli* 'small'; see also Buš. *kengelewoy* 'smallness'. Bast. *kengli* occurs in the lexicalized phrase *angošt kengli*, which is the Bast. name of the little finger.

In Prs. dictionaries, Prs. *kanǰ* is mostly recorded as 'uvula' (DEHX; see also LAZARD 1990a). However, in STEINGASS 1963 s.v., one also finds *kanǰ* 'the little toe' (from *Nezāmolatba*'). If not a misfiling, one may assume in this case a metaphorical association inside the body term terminology, with the little toe (also finger?) equated to the uvula. Since most denominations of the uvula emphasize the smallness of this part, it could also be possible that *kanǰ* 'uvula' is to be referred to the **kan*-group for 'young, small, etc.'.

With reference to Khot. *kaṇaiska*, BAILEY (1979) also quotes Mnǰ. *kandəra* and *kandir åguškīgå* 'little finger'. See also Mnǰ. *k̆āmdər agūšk̆a* (GRJUNBERG 1972) and *kuhnd-r åguškīgå* (MORGENSTIERNE 1966, from BADAXŠI 1960: 75).

It is much likely that Mnǰ. *kandəra* belongs to the same group as Prs. *kam* 'few, little' (Av. *kamna-*, OP *kamna-*, etc.). This is the position of MORGENSTIERNE, who in IIFL-II quotes Mnǰ. *kandəra* (from GAUTHIOT 1916) s.v. *kʸämder*. The question however still remains open.

As far as Prs. *kamin* 'little finger' (STEINGASS 1963) is concerned, DEHX suggests considering it as a misspelling of *kehin* (*angošt*), for which see above, § 1.6.

1.8. Phl. *andak angust* 'little finger' (BAHĀR 1966: 83) contains the MPrs. adj./adv. *andak* 'little; few', continued in Prs. *andak* 'little, few, small' and its several cognates in Iranian.

1.9. Lār. *kaidenû* is the comp./superl. form[276] of Lār.-Ger. *kaidû* 'small', (with an echo-iterative formation *kaidû maidû* 'very small, tiny'). It occurs in the Lār. idiom *kelike-kaidenû* 'little finger'.

Lār. *kaidû* has variants *kaū* and *keve* (ADIB TUSI 1963–1964). Here could also belong Farām. *gedi* 'having a small growth [*kam rošd*]'; SouthKrd. *kada* 'young boy; unacquainted'; Zā. (Siverek) *gidî* 'klein' (HADANK 1932: 156); Tāl. (Langorān) *gada* 'small, minute' (ABDOLI 2001: 205). Nothing can be said about possible connections with the group of MPrs. *kōdak* 'young, small, baby', Prs./Taj. *kudak* 'child', Yγn. *gudik, kudak* 'small child; boy', etc.

---

276 On the ending *-nū* see also above, p. 154.

1.10. In Sogdian, the little finger is named *rinčaku angušt* (SUNDERMANN 2002: 44 no. 59), a phrase containing *rinčaku*, from *rinčăk, rinčē* 'child; small; little; light'; see also *rinčūk* 'child; little; light', *rinčīk* 'small'.

Sgd. *rinčăk* 'small' has several Ir. cognates. However, to which Ir. words it should be connected remains debatable. On the one hand, there are scholars like HENNING (1945: 482 n. 5), GERSHEVITCH (1959: 215, 327) and EMMERICK (1968: 10), who refer *rinčăk* etc. to Av. *raγu-* (Sgd. *ryncwk* < **ranǰuka-*, cf. Av. *raγu-*, *rənǰ-*), and consequently to the IIr. (and IE) words for 'light'/'swift' (EWA II: 423–424; IEW 660–661 **leg^{u}h-*, *leng^{u}h-*). In Iranian, these are Av. *raγu-* 'light; swift' (comp. *rənǰō* [adv.]; superl. *rənǰišta-* 'swiftest'), Man. Prth. *raγ* 'quick; swift', Khot. *rrajsga-* 'swift, light (not heavy)', Khwar. *rnc* 'light (not heavy)', Oss. *ræw, ræwæg* 'light (of weight); swift', Par. *rau, raw* 'quickly' (IIFL-I), Sariq. *rinʒ/c* 'light (of weight), fast (horse)' (EVŠG), Wx. *ranǰg* 'swiftly; lightly' (STEBLIN-KAMENSKY 1999: 459), Semn. *reyka* 'swift', Tāl. *rə(j)* 'fast; swift', Zā. (Siverek, Kur) *ráu* 'schnell' (HADANK 1932: 165–166), to which one may add KurmKrd. *r̠eve-r̠ev* 'swiftly' and *lev* 'swift, fast' in Farāmarzi, a *r-* > *l-* dialect in South-East Iran.

On the other hand, there are scholars who apparently separate the 'small'-line from the 'light/swift'-line, and do not mention Sgd. *rinčăk* as belonging to the latter lexical set (ABAEV [IESOJ], MORGENSTIERNE [EVŠG], STEBLIN-KAMENSKY 1999). In this case, cognates of Sgd. *rinčăk* could only be Pšt. *rangáy*, Man. Prth. *rangas* 'small, short; brief'. They would belong to the Ir. base **rang-* 'to be small' reconstructed by BAILEY (1979) in order to explain Khot. *pārajs-* 'to decrease', *ārraj-* 'to diminuish, shrink'.[277] Of Pšt. *rangáy* 'thin, scanty, shallow, slight, not dense', MORGENSTIERNE states in EVP (s.v. *rōγ*) that it «is prob. not connected with *raghu-* etc., as words belonging to this group are not found in the sense of 'small' etc. (cf. Gr. ἐλακύς) in Indo-Ir.».[278] In fact, there is a lot of IA words for 'small' which may be adduced here; cf. CDIAL 10896 Skt. *laghú-* (RV *raghú-*) 'light' (also Add.). What about Iranian? MORGENSTIERNE's statement is disproved by several Ir. words, which may be added to Sgd. *rinčăk*, Pšt. *rangáy* (also *rangṛáy*), Prth. *rangas* and the Khot. verbs *pārajs-* and *ārraj-*. I will mention them in the following, without entering into details as far as phonetic and/or morphological peculiarities of any single word are concerned:[277a] Šir. *renǰ*

[277] BAILEY 1979 is partially inconsistent in that he mentions the 'swift'-line s.v. *pārajs-* and *ārraj-*, where Sgd. *rinčăk* is also quoted, but not s.v. *rrajsga-* 'swift'.

[277a] Note the striking similarity between the Fārs dialect *renǰ*-type and Sgd. *rinčăk*.

[278] This word has not been included in NEVP.

'small, fine [*deraxt mive-ye renǰ-i dārad* "the tree has small fruits"]; handful [*yek renǰ-i gandom be man dād* "he gave me a handful of corn"]', Kāz. *renǰ* 'small, few; *yek renǰ-i gandom* 'the quantity of corn that may be grasped by a hand; small quantity of corn' (BEHRUZI 2002), Zarq. *renǰ* 'small, fine', Dašt. *renǰ* 'handful, the quantity of things like rice, grain, corn etc. which may be contained in a fist', Abd. *renǰ*, Dav. *rinǰ*, Kal. (Lor) *renǰ* (SALĀMI 2004: 152–153), Ban., Rič., Kal. (Tāǰ.), Mosq. *renǰ* (SALĀMI 2005: 154–155), Dorun., Kor. *renǰ* (SALĀMI 2006: 163) 'handful, fist', Biz. *lek* 'small quantity' (MAZRAᶜTI *et al.* 1995; *semāvar i lek ow pi derä* "in the samovar there is a small quantity of water"), Bard. *riqu* 'small and fine', Fin. *rayg* 'thin and scanty', Jir.-Kahn. *reγenč* 'meagre and emaciated person', SulKrd. *rîwe̱le* 'very thin, skinny'. In Tāleši, *ruk* means 'small' in the dialects of Māsāl (NAWATA 1982: 116), Māsule (LAZARD 1979), Zide and Pare Sar (BAZIN 1981: 276). See also Lāhiǰ. *rīk* 'young boy'; Avarāzān *rikalū* 'small plum' (ADIB TUSI 1963–1964).

HAIM (1992b, s.v. *thin*, in the sense of 'watery, runny'), gives *sabok* as an alternative to Prs. *ābaki*, *kam-māye*, *raqiq*. This means that the concept of LIGHTNESS may be associated in Prs. with that of SMALL DENSITY, offering a motivation for the following Ir. words: Semn., Sang. *row* 'thin, liquid, tender', SouthKrd. *rau* (BĀBĀN 1982, s.v. *ābaki*), KurmKrd. *r̠on* 'dilute, fluid; liquid', Āvarz. *rew* 'soft, dilute' (DEHGHAN 1970), Sirǰ. *row* 'thin, watery (said of a soup thinner than usual)', Zar. *rew* 'thin, dilute' as well as Zar. *laq*, Biz. *läy* (MAZRAᶜTI *et al.* 1995), Ār.-Bidg. *lay, laq*, Bxt. *laγ* etc. 'loose'. I would add here Prs. *leh* 'mashed, crushed', Damāv. *req* 'id.', Bast. *la:h* 'soft and broken up', etc.

LIGHTNESS and QUICKNESS easily overlap: Prs. *sabok* 'light' has also been used in the literary language in the sense of 'fast, swift'. LIGHTNESS and SMALLNESS overlap as well. We have seen some examples above. Witness to this conceptual association in Iranian is born by the semantic range acquired by *sevek̂*, *sevak̂* in (Tāǰ.) Kalāni (Fārs), meaning 'short, small, fine', which corresponds to Prs. *sabok* (and its several cognates). Actually, the name of the little finger in (Tāǰik) Kalāni is *penǰar-e sevek.*[279]

1.11. BADAXŠI (1960: 75) gives *čïṭ ingit* as the little finger name in Iškāšmi and Sangleči. Sangl.. Išk. *čïṭ*, Sgl. *čəṭ* 'small' have an IA origin; cf. **chōṭṭa* 'small' in CDIAL 5071. Sgl. *čəṭ* is also mentioned by MORGENSTIERNE in IIFL-II: 519 with reference to Wx. *čuṭ car-* 'to tear

[279] ° *serek* in SALĀMI 2005: 67 has to be considered as a misprint.

asunder, to be torn'. Wx. *čuṭ* is IA, as well; cf. CDIAL 4965, 4968–70, 5035, 5040, etc. I would also add here Bal. *čaṭ* 'scattered totally; dispersed interely; ruined, destroyed' (see also Br. *čaṭ* 'ruined; scattered').

Par. *čino, činō̈* 'small', which we find in the Par. idiom *aŋgušt-e činō̈/činō̈ γošt* 'little finger' is likewise IA by origin. It belongs to Skt. *cūrṇa-* and cognates (CDIAL 4889).

1.12. Ydγ. *rīza oguščiko* 'small finger' is a lexicalized phrase containing the adjective *rīza* 'small', possibly a Prs. loanword. Prs. *rize* 'small, fine' has several cognates (in many cases, adapted borrowings from Prs.), which are spread almost everywhere in the Iranian plateau.

1.13 In *Gr.Bd.* (4.14-5.3), Ahriman's creation is described as it deserves, i.e., as terrible, rotten and ill-thinking. As least, so it appeared to Ohrmazd, when he saw it. On the contrary, Ohrmazd's creation appeared as vast, profound and intelligent to Ahriman, when he saw it.

In this passage there is a word (4.15) which has been interpreted in different ways. It is an adjective describing Ahriman's creation. NYBERG (1931: 162) reads it as «*nitak* etwa ,in der Tiefe befindlich, wohnend; nach unten gerichtet' [...] Altir. **ni-ta-ka-* zu *ni-*». BAILEY (1933: 2) reads instead *wadag* (*vatak*) and translates 'evil'.[280] Given the adjective *was* 'much, many' used with regard to Ohrmazd's creation, I think that an epithet "small, of no value" for the Ahrimanian one would better fit the rethorical structure of the text.

If a Phl. form *nidag* (or *nitak*?) actually existed, it was certainly not much used in the extant texts. However, a nominal derivative *nidagīh* 'lowliness' could be retraced in *Dk.* VI (E 33, SHAKED 1979: 202–203).[281] This assumed Phl. *nidag* could be related to Phl. *nidom* 'least, smallest'. One could even recognize Modern WIr. cognates, in particular Bxt. (ČLang) *nita* 'small, fine' (also *niteluni* 'a little; small, fine', *nijǰa* 'small'), Šušt. *nit* 'a little', SouthKrd. *niče* 'a little'.

In fact, one could also assume a contamination between different lexical sets conceived as conceptually close. Besides meaning 'a little', Šušt. *nit* also means 'louse'; see also SouthKrd. *nût* 'very new; new-born louse', *notk, notke, notilk* 'new-born louse', KurmKrd. *nûtik*, Āvarz. *nitta*, Dav. *nizg*, Zarq. *nizg, nizgak*, Dašt. *netik, nitak, nečik*, Farām. *nitakoo*, etc. 'new-born

280 Same reading and interpretation in ANKLESARIA 1956: 7.

281 For a possible, different reading and interpretation (*nīdagīh* 'submission', from 'being led'), see SHAKED 1979: 306–307.

louse'. Dašt. *netik, nitak, nečik* is also used as a reference element to emphasize smallness, as is proven by the following sentence: *čišeš mesle nitak-ye* "his eyes are similar to lice", i.e., "his eyes are very small".

Bxt. (ČLang) *nita* 'small, fine' occurs in the ČLang name of the little finger, which is *kelek nita*.

1.14. Taj. *mayda* is a common (literary and dialectal) word for 'small, little'. Though with minor semantic differences, this word is widespread in northern Tajik (see *mayda* 'small (of dimension); little (of tender age), minor; tiny, small (change, of money)' in RASTORGUEVA 1963) and southern Tajik (Kara-Tegin *maydkuk* 'small, tiny' ROZENFEL'D 1982, Badaxš. *mayda* 'child' ŠĀLČI 1991). The form *maydayak* 'very small, very tiny', a derivative of *mayda*, occurs in *čilik-i-maydayak* (KALBĀSI 1995), one of the Taj. labels for the little finger.

Yγn. *mayda(hak)* is a loanword from Tajik. It is a high-frequency word, often used with reference to children. It also occurs in the Yγn. name of the little finger: *maydá páxa* (XROMOV 1972), *maydahak čilik* (MIRZOZODA 2008, s.v. *naxna*).

Cognates of Taj. *mayda* are found elsewhere, though generally used in a restricted number of collocates. In Persian, *meyde* (DEHX, LAZARD 1990a) designates the superfine flour. The bread and a kind of sweet prepared with that quality flour bear the same name. In fact, it is not a 'common' word in Persian, and Persian speakers from Tehran I asked about argued that they have never heard it. In the Persian dialect of Širāz, *meydeh* means 'a rotten fruit, tending to melt'. Sist. *mēda* 'completely ground and softened' is mostly used with reference to flour-like elements, but is also used to describe very fine stitches in tailoring and a good furrow in ploughing the field. The Sist. phrasal verb *mēda kardā*, besides meaning 'to make something very soft', has also the figurative meaning of 'to beat someone and give him a thrashing'.

Prs. *meyde* probably entered the Balochi, Pashto and Parāči lexica; cf. Bal. *mayda* (EBal. *mayδa, mayδaw*) 'fine flour of a very good quality (SAYAD HASHMI 2000, MAYER 1910), 'fine-ground, milled' (ELFENBEIN 1990-II), Pšt. *maydá* 'finely ground flower; superfine flour; fine (of flour, of writing); small (change)', Par. *maida* 'crushed' (IIFL-I). Ur. *maida* 'fine (or the finest) flour or meal' and Si. *maydo* 'fine flour; powder, anything pulverised' seem at first sight Prs. loanwords.

Should one define the semantic core of this word, one could point to the notion of BEING CRUSHED/POWDERED, or BEING MINUTE or BEING SOFT.

From a cognitive point of view, all of these notions may be easily connected with the senses we have seen above for Prs. *meyde* and cognates. TrbHayd. *nerma* 'small; a little of anything', if compared with Prs. *narm* 'soft', bears another witness to the conceptual association between SOFTNESS and SMALLNESS.

Besides Par. *maida* 'crushed', MORGENSTIERNE (IIFL-I) also records Par. *maṛō̈* 'soft', and refers to Skt. *mṛdú-* 'id.' (see CDIAL 10292; EWA II: 372–373). KIEFFER (1979–1980 s.v.) rejects such a comparison and suggests considering Par. *maṛō̈* as «participe passé (= parf.) du v. *maṛ-* employé comme adj, plutôt que < *mṛdu* -». According to MORGENSTIERNE, Par. *maṛ-* 'to rub', Ōrm. *maṛ-* 'to knead, grind' are connected to Skt. *mṛd-* 'to crush'; they are to be considered as loanwords on account of *-ṛ-*. The same holds for Ōrm. *mâṛ* 'flour'. At any rate, Skt. *mṛdú-* 'soft' cannot be separated from Skt. *mṛd-* 'to crush' (EWA II: 386–387, MRAD).

On account of phonetic reasons, Prs. *meyde* could hardly be considered as a direct outcome from OIr. **mṛd-* 'soft', to which probably belong the proper names **Mṛdu-*, **Maṛduniya-* and **Mạrdunika-* (TAVERNIER 2007: 61, 253–254, with literature), trasmitted through Elamite and Babylonian texts. However, the exit of what could have been an original *-ṛd-* could point to a loanword from an Indian language of a cognate word (and this fact justifies the consistent presence of *meyde* in Tajik [*mayda*] and not in Persian of Iran).

1.15. Qm. *kal angošt*, Sang. *kal angošt* (*kal-angošt-u* in AZAMI – WINDFUHR 1972), Lāsg. *qalqalin engošt*, probably Srx. *kil-engošt* and *kule-engošt*,[282] and, in Eastern Iranian, Par. *kel γošt* 'little finger' deserve a special attention.[283]

We have seen above (pp. 107 ff.) some Ir. *kal*-forms meaning 'big' (and by a semantic extension 'male'), which concur in forming lexicalized phrases designating the thumb. Qm. *kal*, Sang. *kal* etc., occurring in denominations for the little finger, should obviously be something different, because a label depicting the little finger as a "big finger" would not be felt cognitively grounded and in no way accepted. Contrast as an associative principle is by far the less important among the associative principles involved in lexical change (BLANK 2001: 14). The only case we have met with so far is the EBal. idiom *šābāš murdānaγ* 'forefinger' (see above, p. 123). No other instance I am able to put

282 But see also below, fn. 168.

283 See also Roš. *khal-lakak* 'ringfinger', mentioned above p. 147.

forward, as far as Ir. designations of body parts relying on this principle. Therefore, it is better to go in search for something else.

Looking for it, we find a lexical element linking Fārs-Lārestān dialects and some dialects spoken in North Iran, which seems to come up with our expectations. In the coastal area south of Fārs, *kal* means 'child, son'. This information is given by BEHRUZI (1969), who provides the following example: *in bačče kal-e ali-st* "this child is Ali's son", and confirmed by HAMIDI (2001), cf. Buš. *kal* (Tangestāni *kelak*) 'child, son', Dašt. *kelak, keleku*[284] 'boy, little boy'. See also Mās. *käläk* 'Sohn' (MANN 1909), Kāz. *kalaku* 'small son, boy' (BEHRUZI 2002), Zarq. *kalaku, karaku*, used as a term of address for babies, Farām. *kalak* 'child' and Bast. *ka:la:k* 'little child', which find correspondences in Māz. *kel* 'small, child', *kele* 'child', Tāl. *kela* 'daughter; girl', IrĀz. *kille*, (Šā) *kila*, (GL) *kelleg*, (Xu) *kêla* 'girl' (ABDOLI 2001: 234).[285] Ham. *kal* 'youth, puberty' could probably be added here. EILERS (1974: 330 n. 59a) mentions the forms *kalak* 'Kleinigkeit, Unwichtiges' and *kalaki* 'leichtes Mädchen, Dirne', both labelled by him as Persian.

Ōrm. *klân* 'son', *klanâk* 'boy', for which MORGENSTIERNE (IIFL-I: 398) suggested a doubtful connection with Krd. *kurr* 'son', could belong here. Note also *kaldukak* 'child, son' in the Taj. dial. spoken by the Čistāniha, living in Uzbekistan (MAHMUDOV 2001: 45). I am tempted to include here *kal-*, a sort of prefix for nominal derivation, used in a few Eastern Prs. varieties, viz. Sistāni and Birǰandi. This is "a prefix which gives the meaning of 'similar to, along the lines of', or 'uncomplete' or 'half-'" (REZĀI 1998); see e.g. Birǰ. *kalexoš(k)* 'a bit dry, more or less dry' and Sist. *kala koš* 'half-killed' (Sist. *kala* 'half-'). The position of Buš. *kalil* 'small', used as a term of endearment for children, is doubtful; it could also be considered as an alteration of Prs. *qalil* 'little, few, scanty' (< Ar.).

---

[284] Dašt. *keleku*, beside being a *u*-derivative from *kelak*, is also its determined form; therefore, it may be understood both as 'boy' and 'that boy'.

[285] Mās. *käläk* is problematically quoted by CHRISTENSEN – BARR 1939 s.v. KrmnšKrd. *kälgâ* 'junger Faselstier, noch nicht Arbeit getan, zur Zucht' («Ob Fârs M. *käläk* ,Sohn' [...] auch hinzugehört, ist fraglich»). This perplexity seems quite justified. In fact, there are different, deep-rooted groups of words in Iranian, phonetically similar to (and probably sometimes intersecting with) each other, which I think may be outlined as follows: (1) *kal*-words for 'big/male' we have seen above, including those referring to male (general adult; often horned) animals, such as bulls, buffalos or billy goats; (2) *kal*-words for 'bald, bald-headed' (see FILIPPONE 2006: 367 f.), including words referring to hornless animals, i.e. hornless goats or the like; (3) *kal*-words for 'small' (commented on in the main text).

All this considered, Sang. *kal angošt* etc. can be interpreted as "the small/young finger", according to a recurrent iconomastic pattern.

It is not clear if we should consider the above mentioned *kal*-forms for 'small' as connected to Prs. *kal* 'short', recorded in traditional dictionaries (but not consistently; see DEHX). Prs. *kal* (see also Taj. *kalta* 'docktailed', Yγn. *kalta* 'short' MIRZOZODA – QOSIMI 1995) could be a variant of Prs. *kol* 'short', which has several cognates widespread mainly in WIr. A good collection is in REZĀZĀDE MALEK 1973. One could also ascribe Srx. *kil-engošt* and *kule-engošt* (mentioned above, p. 166) to the *kol*-type and intend it as 'the short finger', on the basis of the same conceptualization pattern which has produced Knd. *penǰe-y kolulu* and Qasr. *kol angušd* 'little finger'.

1.16. Dusir. *penǰe-y lošu* is one of the little finger names recorded in Fārs. It contains an adj. base (Dusir. *loš* 'small'), which appears quite isolated and requires further investigation.

2. Many (if not the majority) of the little finger names discussed at §§ 1.1–1.15, which for the sake of convenience we may simply refer to as the "small-finger" labels, are actually figurative expressions, which evoke the image of a finger conceptualized as a child. As we have seen above, to the little finger, mothers, fathers or brothers may also be attributed.

All this considered, Biz. *māmāčelīk* (an alternative to *čelīk* 'little finger') and Qohr. *māne küliče* 'little finger', which may look like fitting names for the ring finger (see "the mother of the little finger" pattern above, p. 147), are difficult to explain. Once lost the consciousness of the original iconym, the name of a particular finger (in this case, the ring finger) could have been used for another finger. What is strange, however, is that both expressions appear still transparent in their structure; cf. Qohr. *māne*, Biz. *mama* 'mother'. Possibly, we have to do here with the phenomenon common in Iranian (and elsewhere), according to which a same address term is used as a cross-reference term between two different generational levels (e.g., mother/father towards their children and *vice versa*). But this hypothesis seems not to be fully convincing.

Besides lucky little fingers, which can rely on mothers, there are also poor, "lacking parents" fingers, as is the case with Taj. *angušt-i yatimak*. The "orphan-finger" iconomastic pattern is also found in Osmanli Turk., see *öksüz parmak* 'lit. le doigt sans mère' (ERDAL 1981 : 124).[286]

[286] Note, however, that in REDHOUSE 1968 *öksüz parmak* is 'ring finger'.

3. The metonymical process FINGER → LITTLE FINGER is a very frequent associative process.[287] There are languages in which a single word maintains its general meaning ('finger') and also acquires a specialized one ('little finger'). Instances in Iranian are Voniš. *uŋguss,*[288] Kāz. *angol*, and SouthKrd. *pil* (recorded by SAFIZĀDE 2001 as 'finger' and 'little finger'). There are languages in which the word for 'little finger' shows a semasiological link with words for 'finger' in different but related languages. As for Iranian, compare Keš. *aŋgulī* 'little finger', contrasting with *aŋguš* 'finger'.

To the *kelk*-group 'finger',[289] the following labels for 'little finger' are connected: Prs. *kelik, kalik, kelek, kelikak,*[290] Taj. *kilik*, Birǰ. *kalikk*, Mašh. *kelyk*, Qasr. *kelikak angušd*, Šušt. *kelek* ('finger; sometimes little finger'), Bxt. (Behdārvandi) *kelek* (SĀDEQI 2000: 61),[291] Par. *kilk γušt* (IIFL-I) with *kilk* to be compared with Par. *kelk* 'finger'.

Analogously, to the *kelič*-group 'finger',[292] one may connect the following labels for 'little finger': Prs. *keličak, kelanǰ(ak)*, Taj. *kiličak*, (Fārs dialects) Šir. *kelenǰ* (also 'finger'),[293] Zarq. *kelenǰ,* Sarv. *kilič*, Gurkāni *keliǰak* (JA^{c}FARI DEHAQI 2002: 151), Kuz. *kâlenǰak*, Dahl. *penǰe-y k̂eriček̂*, Gorgn. *penǰe-y k̂elič*, Gavk. *kelīč*, Baliā. *k̂elič* (also 'finger'), KurmKrd. *qilîç'k, qilîncek*; *tilîya qilîç'ke, qilîçane, qilînceke* (also *qilîcan* RIZGAR 1993), SouthKrd. *qilîč, qilîčân, qil̲înǰ, qilînǰâk* (EBRĀHIMPUR 1994b, s.v. *angošt*: *dipila qlîčî*; *qilînǰik*), Zā. (Biǰaq) *qalânǰik* (HADANK 1932: 218), Bxt. *kelič* (LORIMER 1922 *kulīč*[294]), Šušt. *qālič*. In Central Iran, we find Rāv. *keličū*, Del. *γalīčae*, Xur. *kelēč* (*kleič* FARAHVAŠI 1976), Nāi. *engolī keličču* (LECOQ 2002 *kiliči*), Ār.-Bidg. *kēliǰ* (also 'small') and *əgüškliǰ*, Gz. *engolī kulūčī*, ZorYzd. (*angušt-i*) *kilīčōg* (*angošt-e kiliči* AFŠĀR 1989), Yzd-JPrs. *kiliči*.

---

[287] On 'finger' → 'little finger' in Turkish, see ERDAL 1981: 125.

[288] But see above, p. 54.

[289] Cf. above, pp. 63 f.

[290] Prs. speakers from Tehran I consulted, recognized these Prs. words as belonging to the literary register, but only with the meaning of 'finger' (and not 'little finger').

[291] In his review to VAHMAN – ASATRIAN 1987, SĀDEQI (2000: 59–61) provides a list of discordances between the Bxt. words gathered by LORIMER and those personally collected by him from a (Behdārvandi) Bxt. speaker. Among them, note *kelek* 'little finger' instead of LORIMER's *kulīč* 'id.'.

[292] Cf. above, pp. 64 f.

[293] See also above p. 64, fn. 60.

[294] See also above, fn. 291.

To these forms, add Prs. *kābleǰ, kābliǰ, kāblič, kāluǰ, kāluč* (all unknown to Prs. speakers of Tehran I consulted) and Taj. *kobliǰ*.

Note also Khwar. *k'lwǰ* 'little finger' (YÜCE – BENZING 1985).[295] Bal. (?) *kābalošk* 'little finger', recorded by the author of an unpublished dictionary (NAGUMAN n.d; SouthBal.?) is in all probability a (Eastern) Prs. word adapted to Balochi.

In Kermān and adjacent areas, one finds Kerm. (*angošte/nāxune) kāčilu* or *kāčil*, Bard., Sirj. *kāčilu* and probably also *xaǰilek* which ŽUKOVSKIJ (1922: 110) provides as the name of the little finger in Abdui, a Krd. variety spoken in a small village in Fārs. This latter reminds SouthKrd. *qiǰîlik* 'little finger'.

Should we consider this group of words as belonging to the *kal* ('small')-forms, instead of resorting to the *kelk*-type and consequently to the FINGER / LITTLE FINGER = STICK associative pattern we have suggested above? Mentioning Prs. *kalak* 'Kleinigkeit, Unwichtiges', EILERS (1974: 330 n. 59a) advances the hypothesis of its possible connection with Prs. *kelek, kelanǰ(ak)* 'little finger'. This sounds as possible, also in the light of Anār. *kiliču*, Ardest. *kiličči* 'very small', Varz. *keleču* 'small', Ār.-Bidg. *kēliǰ* 'small' (besides 'little finger'). Or should we rather presume that a metathesis has occurred in forms similar to Prs. *kučulu* (as doubtfullly suggested by EILERS (1979) as regards Gz. *kulūčī* in *engolī kulūčī*)?

Frankly, I think it is very hard to take a clear stand on this issue, and probably many factors have combined to create this complicated situation. Large margins for doubts remain.

One may relate Biz. *čelīk*, Yγn. (Prs. lw.) *čīlīk* 'little finger' to dial. Taj. *čilik* 'finger' (see above p. 65). Lexicographers are somehow contradictory as far as Prs. *čelk* is concerned. The definitions gathered in DEHX sound as follows: 'little finger [*xenser; angošt-e kučak*]'; 'the finger of the hand which is between the middle finger [*angošt-e vasati*] and the ring finger [*benser*]';[296] 'ring finger [*angošt-e benser*]' and 'little finger [*kučaktarin angošt-e dast*]'. In FF *čelk* is recorded as 'middle finger; ring finger', in STEINGASS 1963 as 'little finger'. The word was unknown to Prs. speakers of Tehran I consulted on the matter.[297]

[295] I thank Mauro MAGGI for having pointed out to me this Khwar. word.

[296] Sic! *benser* is probably DEHXODĀ's oversight for *xenser*.

[297] See also above, p. 155.

KurmKrd. *tilî*, a figurative expression for 'finger' having its conceptual source in the botanical domain,[298] finds a partial correspondence in Lo. *kalak-e tīla* (UNVALA 1958: 14) 'little finger'. TurkĀz. *tīl*, seemingly a measure of length corresponding to a little finger ([*az nuk-e angošt-e kučak tā kaf-e dast*]), could be an Ir. lw. belonging here.

4. Ordinary derivative suffixes conveying the notion of SMALLNESS, added to words for 'finger', change them into 'little finger'. This happens in Persian, where *angošt* and *angol* have produced *angoštak* and *angolak* 'little finger', in Tajik, where *angušt* and *lela* 'finger' have become *anguštak* and *lelača* 'little finger', and in the Tajik dialect of Kara-Tegin, where *lik* 'finger' contrasts with *likak, likək* 'little finger' (ROZENFEL'D 1982). Šγn. *likak* (BADAXŠI 1960: 75), *lakak, lakak angiẋt*, Baǰ. *lakak ingaẋt* 'little finger' are probably Taj. borrowings. In Kābuli, *kelkak* 'little finger' derives from *kelk* 'finger' (FARHÂDI 1955: 104). Similarly, Šir. *angolak*, Kāz. *angolak* (BEHRUZI 2002) and Lir.-Dil. *angûlak* 'little finger' derive from *angol/angûl* 'finger'.

Haz. *čilkak* 'little finger' presupposes a *čil(i)k* 'finger', not recorded in the Haz. sources available to me (but documented in dial. Tajik). It could also be interpreted as a secondary derivation from Haz. (< Prs./Taj.) **čilk* 'little finger' (see Prs. *čelk* above p. 170).

5. Syllabic iteration is a lexicalization device with an ideophonic value. Lexical items created reduplicating a syllable expressively evoke the feelings and emotions of people towards the relevant referents, implying a strong involvement of human perception. SMALLNESS is one of the concept which may be evoked by such a device.[299] With reference to the little finger, we may quote Bal. *čūč*, (mostly EBal.) *čīč, čīnč* and the several derivatives *čūčī, čūčū, čūčūk, čūčik, čīčuk, čūčag, čūčkul, čīčkul, čičkur* (*lankuk*), *čūnčī mačūnčī, čīnčuk, čīnčuko, čīčako*, all variants (and/or derivatives) – with minor differences – of a common *č*V*č*(V) pattern.[300] Br. *čīčak, čīčal, čič-hōr* are with a good probability borrowed directly from Bal. (cf. ROSSI 1979: F36) , even if this lexical pattern for 'little finger' should be considered as an areal lexical feature. As regards IA, cf. Sir. *chīchī*, Si. *chīch*[a]. Phonetic similarity is also shown by some Turk. labels, such as TurkĀz. *čečələ*, Kyrgyz *činčilaq*, Uzbek *žimžiloq*, *čimčaloq*

---

298 Cf. above p. 66.

299 A few examples are available in FILIPPONE 1995: 51 ff.

300 For a more detailed dialectal distribution of these forms see FILIPPONE 2000–2003: 69.

(ABDURAXMANOV 1954),[301] to which Yγn. *činčilak* 'little finger' (*činčilik* 'finger' in MIRZOZODA 2008), Taj. *čimčilok* 'finger' could be related.[302]

The *čVč(V)/ǰVǰ(V)* pattern for naming small things of different kinds seems to be highly productive and sometimes it is very difficult to say which is the primary sense among the many senses that a single term of this series might have.[303] Instances of this pattern in Iranian are Xor. *čūča* 'small; infant', *čūčagak* 'small, very small', TrbHayd. *čuča* 'small child', Fārsivāni *čuč* 'small of animal' (MAHMUDOV 2001), Bal. *čūčag* 'small; child, baby' (SAYAD HASHMI 2000), Ir.Bal. (Sarhaddi) *čūčok* 'chick' (AYYUBI 2002), KurmKrd. *ç'ûç'ik* 'small, little; child', *ç'îç'ik* 'small amount, little bit', etc., Prs. *ǰuǰe* 'chicken', Bādr. *ǰiǰ* 'small', Qm. *ǰiǰil* 'small', Tāl. *ǰinǰili* 'very small, minute, tiny' (ABDOLI 2001) and many, many others. Several terms belonging to the body part lexicon have been produced by means of this lexical device. Besides little fingers, one also find nipples, parts of the female genital organs, uvulas, etc.; they will be treated in detail on another occasion.

A *tVt(V)*-pattern for 'little finger' links Gorāni, Southern/Central Kurdish and Lori. Cf. SorKrd. *pence tūta* (HAKIM – GAUTHIER 1993),[304] *qamkî tûteḻe* (KURDOEV – JUSUPOVA 1983), SulKrd. *pencetûte*, SouthKrd. *angustî/kilka/panǰa tûta* (SAFIZĀDE 2001), (Krmnš.) *kelek tuta*; *tutela*, (Garr.) *kelik e tûtä*, Gor. (Gahw.) *kilík i tûtä*,[305] (Talahed.) *kelek tüta*, Lak. *keĺek tuita*, Lo. *kelek tita*, (Xorramābād) *tîta* (HASURI 1964: 24).

The *tVt(V)*-pattern similarly produces many Ir. designations for affectively connoted referents. A few instances are provided in FILIPPONE 1995: 54 ff.; to them add Zā. *tūt* 'child', Dav. *titi*, Dašt. *titi* 'baby, small child', Tehr. *titiš* 'small', Lo. *tita* 'small and nice' (ADIB TUSI 1963–1964), etc.

---

301 As an instance of Turk. little finger labels styled «de nature expressive», ERDAL (1981: 122) quotes Old Turk. *çıçamuq* and suggests interpreting it as «un dérivé du verb qui se réfère à la décharge des excréments: évidemment, le créateur du terme a pensé à l'incontinence des petits enfants». However, one should remind that the sublexicon related to excrements, especially that used with/by children, is in all languages affected by expressive labels created by iterating syllables (cf. for example Engl. *whee-whee*; *pooh-pooh* etc.). Possibly, the Turk. terms for 'little finger' and 'act of urinating' share the same syllabic pattern, having no other conceptual connection.

302 See also above, pp. 66, 89.

303 Cf. KORN 2005: 293 fn. 45 (« *čūčū* etc. can be specialisations of *čūčag* "child, baby; tiny" [...] which might also be of onomatopoetic origin»).

304 S.v. *doigt* (petit doigt); *pencey tûne* ibid. s.v. *auriculaire* should be considered as a misprint.

305 So rightly emended by CHRISTENSEN – BARR (1939: 305) instead of *kilik-i sûtä* in HADANK 1930: 449.

According to MORGENSTIERNE (1932a: 40), EBal. *kūko*, recorded as 'little finger' in HETU RAM 1898 and as 'finger' in MAYER 1910, is a IA loanword; cf. Si. *kōkō* 'small pin, nail', to which also add AfγPrs. *kūka* 'small pin'. Having found no confirmation of this Bal. word in my fieldwork, I am not in a position to say where and in what sense it is (or was) used. However, it seems reasonable enough to recall here Min. *kukal*, Bšk. *kukalu* 'little finger' (G. BARBERA p.c.), Fin. *kūkaley* 'little finger' (but also 'the smallest child in a family') and envisage a pattern *k*V*k(*V*)*, which may also explain Lār. *kokol* (*kakal* in ADIB TUSI 1963–1964) 'small, tiny', Pšt. *kokáy* 'boy'[306], etc.

One could perhaps interpret in this light even MPrs. *kūk* 'small, short', so far explained as < **kau-ka-*.[307] It may probably also be traced back in a proper name from Achaemenid time (see **Kūka-* 'small, little' in TAVERNIER 2007: 234). In EIr., one could add Ydγ. *kūk^{y}a* 'short'.

An iterative process, with an expressive value, also explains *guluguluy penǰa*, the (isolated) Korš. name of the little finger.

7. The little finger's position seems not to have played a significant role in the naming process. However, we may mention at least a couple of labels which find their motivation in this parameter. These are Prs. *angošt-e panǰom* (DEHX), lit. 'the fifth finger' and Lāsg. *kenārin engošt*, which places emphasis on the side position of this finger, perceived as a "lateral finger".[308]

As for Phl. *pas angust*, lit. 'the behind-finger', given as 'little finger' in ABRAMJAN 1965: 5 (*axar angušt*), a few comments have been offered above, p. 130.

8. A Prs. name for 'little finger', felt as fairly appropriate to a formal register, is *xenser, xensar*, also occurring in Tajik (*angušt-i xinsir*). This is an Ar. loanword; cf. Ar. *xinṣir*, Syr. *ḥeṣra*, Mand. *hiṣra* etc., which belong to a Sem. base «connected or contaminated with Sem. **ḫṣr* 'to be short'» (MILITAREV – KOGAN 2000: no. 134).

9. There is still a couple of labels to be discussed, which appear to be isolated and/or very hard to classify.

---

[306] «Cf. 'rustic' Urdu *khokha* m. 'small', particularly, 'a little child, a boy' [E]», NEVP.

[307] On possible outcomes of the IIr. base **kau-* see also above, p. 151.

[308] Compare Lāsg. *kenārin engošt* with Yzγ. *kəranai γ^{w}ax̌t*, which, however, refers to both 'forefinger' and 'ring finger'; see above p. 129.

SouthKrd. *mît* 'little finger' depicts this finger as a small protuberance. It is an "affective" word, whose cognates are used in the anatomical lexicon to designate the clytoris or similar small parts. Cf. SouthKrd. *mîtk, mîtke, mîtoḻ, mîṯole*, Sist. *mitt*, Birǰ. *mott*, Bal. (Noške; SAYAD HASHMI 2000) *miṭṭ(ik),* (Turbat) *mīčuk* 'clytoris' ('uvula' in Irānšahr, Sarāwāni). See also Br. *miṭṭ* 'clitoris' (ELFENBEIN 1983b).

Roš. *bilisak ingaxt* and Baǰ. *bilīsak ingaxt* could be grounded on a metaphorical association linking the finger with an entomological element, if *bilisak* is the same *bilisak* 'dragonfly' which we find in Rošanī. Roš. *l^e lisak iŋgaxt* (SKÖLD 1936: 186) might be a misprinting or a mishearing of *bilisak ingaxt*; however, it might also be a different, phonosymbolic name, based on syllabic iteration (/V/V-pattern).

Prs. *karišak* 'little finger', recorded by lexicographers but apparently unknown to Iranian Prs. speakers, could be a figurative label which equates the finger to a small, just hatched chick (see DEHX in two different headwords). If so, an analogy could be found in Turkish: see *serçe parmaq* 'the little finger or the little toe' with *serçe* 'sparrow; any small bird'. One cannot exclude, however, that *karišak* in Prs. dictionaries results from a misspelling/misreading of other forms, such as *keličak*, etc.

For the following little finger names, I have no suggestion at all. They are: KurmKrd. *tilîya başikan*; Dav. (*pinǰe-y*) *gârek*; Haz. *ašunan* (DULLING 1973); Tāti (Apšeron) *qilat* (GRJUNBERG 1963: 117).

Pashto and Kurdish seem to have in common a prefix-like element (*bar-*), which, prefixed to terms for 'finger', would produce names for the little finger. Cf. Pšt. *bargúta* (*bargwə́ta* QALANDAR MOMAND – SEHRAYI 1994) 'little finger', as contrasted to Pšt. *gúta* 'finger'; KurmKrd. (*tilyâ*) *barkilîčk* 'little finger' (SAFIZĀDE 2001), as contrasted to the *kelič*-type 'finger'. How could this be explained? Has Krd. *bar-* in *barkilîčk* something to do with Kal.-Adb. *bärî, berî* 'etwas', Mukri *birêk* 'ein wenig' etc. recorded (but defined "unklar") by CHRISTENSEN – BARR (1939: 466)?

WORD INDEX

1. Iranian languages and dialects

MINĀBI

MOSQĀNI

MUNJI

NAQUSĀNI

NĀINI (CENTRAL DIAL.)

PERSIAN OF AFGHANISTAN

2. Non-Iranian Languages